TANTRA: *The Yoga of Sex*

TANTRA: *The Yoga of Sex*

OMAR V. GARRISON

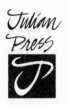

Published by The Julian Press, Inc.,
a division of the Crown Publishing Group,
One Park Avenue, New York, New York 10016.
Published simultaneously in Canada by
General Publishing Company, Limited.

Manufactured in the United States of America

Library of Congress Cataloging in Publication Data
Garrison, Omar V.
Tantra: the yoga of sex by Omar V. Garrison.
New York, Julian Press, 1964.
Bibliography: p. 239–240.

1. Yoga   2. Tantrism.   I. Title.

B132.Y6G35   181.45   64-22230

ISBN 0-517-54947-6 (cloth)
ISBN 0-517-54948-4 (paper)

10   9   8   7   6   5   4   3   2   1

1983 Edition

For W.W.

Contents

Preface

As a medical man who has practiced gynecology and psychosomatic medicine for more than twenty years and
who has had to treat frigidity and impotence, and other
sexual problems of many men and women who came to
me for help, I can say with conviction that never before
have I examined a text that presents the sexual union of
humans and the preliminary relationships leading up to
that goal as lovingly, beautifully and as hopefully as
The Yoga of Sex.

In our times we seem to have made more progress in
coming face to face with our sexuality than in the im-

mediately preceding periods. The work of Sigmund Freud and his followers has encouraged the scientific study of sexual taboos and other aspects of social living which had tended to identify the sex life of humans as obscene, degrading and minimizing; to be conducted in dark seclusion in shame. Their effort has been responsible for a great improvement in the more natural and dignified appreciation of the sex function.

Because of this, modern psychiatrists, physicians, ministers and others whose responsibility is the dissemination of learning, have been teaching the healthful, hygienic-scientific shamefree approach to sexual relationships. They have even gone farther along the road by studying the various physical methods of achieving pleasure in the sex act and have developed manuals to dispel biological ignorance and to aid individuals to achieve sex pleasure.

These may well be important steps in the right direction but, as we know, the sexual relationship is also an emotional one and very subjective. It has to be felt as a flow, as part of living and being, rather than only as a lesson learned which will be marked by a teacher for percentage ratings. And we must also consider the fact that for many who have been reared in traditions where the religious plays a signal role, the concept of rational, hygienic sex education is not initially acceptable; involuntarily they tend to withdraw from such procedures. Even when they seem to accept the new freedom and teaching, when they attempt to apply this methodology, because of some seeming inner incompatibility they tend to become rigid and automatonlike, and another type of frustration is born. For such persons, as well as many others who may not manifest identical symptoms, the awareness that the sex act can be loving, beautiful and holy (not merely in the institutional sense but in terms of a dynamic and expanding universe) is an inspiring and liberating force leading to a greater sense of personal security and more natural human function. And it is not strange when such a sexual transformation occurs that a similar liberation and advance is experienced in other areas of a person's existence.

Modern science, in its eagerness to absorb complete information about the world we live in and to use this knowledge to advance mankind, has been inclined to overly departmentalize and to separate in their studies both creatures and things from their nature and development. In the area of sex this has led to a stage where too many teachers seem to view sex as though it was something that takes place mechanically on purely a rational plane. This error is transmitted to the pupils who proceed to perform the sex role as taught, but in spite of this, wind up without satisfaction and with the feeling of having failed.

In *The Yoga of Sex* the sexual relationship of the male and female is perceived as an integral part of living out the human design and a stage of evolutionary development moving towards a more advanced humankind. Love-Tenderness-Respect-Dignity and the Holy are recognized a part of mankind as much as are his more obvious physical attributes. The female is not less than the male; one does not antagonize the other—but both seek and achieve a unity which reflects the deeper, fuller and higher joys of living. And *The Yoga of Sex* provides training and discipline to prepare for this union since, as their teachers believe, each step of the way is connected to the goal, each step as meaningful, each step as vital and so, there is a continuity and a wholeness.

The breathing exercises described in this book are an important part of the discipline and are unusually healthful and helpful. Followed regularly, as directed, they are both relaxing and invigorating. The quality of relaxation is non-soporific and the reader will discover sources of self-energy available, of which there was no previous awareness. Those who may previously have viewed themselves as unduly passive in the sexual role, will find the desire and ability to actively participate in whatever role is in order.

The Yoga of Sex is based on ancient Tantric wisdom. Tantra Yoga is the only Yoga which comes to grips with human sexuality. One of the major criticisms of Yoga by Western scholars has been the emphasis on celibacy and the seeming disregard of the world in which we live, which to the Western mind and culture represents a rejection of our present existence. Tantra Yoga regards the present as meaningful and as the only means of achieving tomorrow. This knowledge, according to historians, originally was born in India, but whether it was born in India or was brought from some other early highly developed civilization, what is more important is its truly scientific character. These ancients had a view and an understanding of man which, when added and connected to our Western practical approach and development, can add to our stature, increase our ability to perceive and give us a higher purpose and meaning for living. These concepts provide something we seem desperately to lack, that we seek to satisfy in the acquisition of more and more things—in power over others which we do not know how to use—and instead provides us with the means to quiet the frustration of not knowing who we are. It offers joy to replace confusion, hope to replace despair.

I cannot conceive of any reasonable, intelligent, sensitive person reading this work not benefitting from its good sense, its many elements of scientific validity and the vision of a more beautiful and meaningful mankind.

WILLIAM S. KROGER, M.D.

Los Angeles, Calif.
August 1964

> "As one falls on the ground, one must lift oneself
> by aid of the ground."
>
> —*Kularnava Tantra*

Introduction

This book, which will reveal to you some of the closely
guarded secrets of a little-known branch of yoga, was
written with a two-fold purpose in mind.

First was the aim of presenting for the first time in
an easy-to-understand text, the basic philosophy and disciplines of Tantra, a yogic tradition compatible with the
Western way of life.

Second was the desire to place in the hands of sincere
and open-minded readers a means of changing their sex
life from boredom, maladjustment and sensuality into
a sacrament.

The ancient Hindu texts, upon which the practice of Tantra Yoga is based, assert that we today are living in the final years of a debased *yuga* or age—the Age of Kali. They contend that only by laying hold of the power inherent in sex force can we find the creative energy to ascend to spiritual liberation.

A system valid for all peoples

Moreover, they hold that the Shastra (body of literature) which teaches this mystic science is valid for all peoples of the world, and is not limited to Hindus, Tibetans, or to any exclusive group.

They recognize the beauty and truth of transcendental thought in other systems of yoga; but they realistically declare that the ascetic demands made upon the aspirant by such systems render them wholly impractical—indeed, dangerous—for the mass of people.

Strongly supporting this view is the fact that during the past fifty years, scores of swamis and religious teachers have come to the West from India, expounding various spiritual disciplines based upon renunciation of the world as we know it. Almost without exception, they have taught that escape from our present degraded existence into higher realms of being is to be achieved only by rejection of sensual experience, and by means of difficult austerities.

Yet the followers of these systems of self-culture have scarcely become adepts of the kind envisioned by Shankara and Ramanuja. They have come nowhere near achieving the yogic powers said to be the inevitable fruits of such practices.

These include such things as the ability to become "light as cotton wool and fly through the skies"; to know others' thoughts, to become invisible in a crowd, to know the exact time of one's death, and so on.

Any impartial observer who measures results against such claims must sadly conclude that, for our age, these yogas offer little other than intellectual interest or negative inspiration.

The four cycles

Tantrik texts, both Hindu and Buddhist, declare from the outset that each *yuga* or vast cycle of time permeates with its particular influences not only human beings, but everything, organic or inorganic, in the universe.

During *satya yuga*, the golden age before man's spiritual powers began to decline, these influences were of the highest order. Men, who were physical as well as spiritual giants, enjoyed a prolonged lifespan. The Shastra describes them as truthful, honest, kind, pure in heart; free of vanity, greed, anger and lust.

As in the Christian heaven, where "they neither marry nor are given in marriage," so in the first age, sexual union was unknown. Children, we are told, came into being through fervent and loving wish.

In the next and slightly lower age—*treta yuga*—procreation was accomplished by touch. The practice of "high" yoga, as prescribed in the Vedic texts, was still known, although it had become more difficult. The race of man was smaller of stature, both physically and spiritually. Moreover, human lifespan became shorter.

In the third age on the descending scale, called the *dvapara yuga,* men and women began to copulate as they do in our age. At the same time, their physical stature decreased by one half what it had been during the *satya yuga.* They lived only one tenth as long. Their spiritual powers likewise declined sharply, so that they could no longer follow their dharma. That is, "men were no longer able, by Vedic practices, to accomplish their desires."

To them a new scripture, suited to their needs, was given. These texts were called the Puranas.

With the fulfillment and passing away of the third cycle, our own age, fourth and lowest of all, emerged.

A manual of sexual liberation

Tantrik literature describes it as a time of great striving and tribulation; of deceit and sorrow. The practices and rites of the *satya yuga* have long since been abandoned, except in text, for they are no longer practicable. We are too feeble, too much the creatures of our senses to undertake the austerities of self-discipline as spelled out in the prime Vedic scriptures. For us a different manual of liberation has been provided—the Tantras.

In the Mahanirvana Tantra, men of our age are described as "without restraint; maddened with pride, ever given over to sinful acts; lustful, gluttonous, cruel, heartless, harsh of speech, deceitful, short-lived."

The Vishnu Purana likewise describes the life of our age with amazing accuracy. It declares that men will know they have entered the Kali Age "when society reaches a stage where property confers rank, wealth becomes the only source of virtue, passion the sole bond of union between husband and wife, falsehood the source of success in life, sex the only means of enjoyment, and when outer trappings are confused with inner religion."

This is not to say that we pygmies of the Kali Age have not progressed intellectually. A billion years of evolution have endowed the three-pound mass of gray matter in our skulls with an amazing power to transform the world around us.

But this ability to perform the highest levels of integration; to screen, codify, condense, edit and remember the infinite number of stimuli entering the reticular system, is not a spiritual process except in an oblique way. It is not the high calling to which the Vedic scriptures addressed themselves.

On the contrary, Tantrik teachers imply that it is precisely this bewildering activity that will eventually mechanize, brutalize, and destroy mankind.

The mystical marriage of God and Man

With the present spiritual state of man in mind, therefore, the early Tantrik texts make no attempt to philosophize in the grand and elaborate manner of many of the Indian schools. Rather, the treatises set forth at once those concrete details needed as a guide leading us toward the harmonious union of opposing forces within ourselves, that is, towards the Mystical Marriage of God and man.

Tantra provides each seeker with a manual (suited to his individual needs) for embarking upon the adventure of self-exploration and self-conquest.

While in every instance the aim is the same—reintegration of opposite polarities within the disciple's own body—the various disciplines formulated for accomplishing this end differ among the manifold esoteric traditions of Tantrism.

Moreover, there are what might be called higher and lower traditions. The texts upon which these diverse schools base their teachings are numerous and often recondite. Many have been lost altogether. Others remain in extremely fragmentary and sometimes altered form. Some are kept closely guarded by the sects possessing them.

Vidya Gupta—a secret doctrine

In several important ways, Tantrism is and must remain a secret doctrine (vidya gupta), imparted only by word of mouth from guru to disciple. Even some of the written scriptures available to us are intelligible only to those who hold the key to their symbolism and inner meanings.

It is not surprising, therefore, that up to the present time, only tangential and generalized popular accounts of the system have appeared in America. Even these, with one or two notable exceptions, have dwelt upon the more sensational and least understood aspects of the subject.

A yoga that has been roundly denounced by Orthodox Hindus at home, and repudiated by them abroad, is not likely to find easy acceptance in alien cultures.

Nevertheless, those who have made an honest effort to probe the depths of this profound doctrine, have found in it a spiritual dynamic better suited to the needs of the ordinary man than any offered by Vedic purists.

The disciplines offered in the following pages have been, in some respects, modified to meet requirements of the Western student, whose environment and way of life are different from those of the Hindu or Tibetan aspirant.

These exercises and rituals were adapted from traditional formulas by a Bengali guru, who is both a successful man of the world and an adherent of Tantra Shastra.

The present work is in no sense a complete exposition of Tantrism. Rather, it is concerned largely with that portion of it known as Vamachara.

Foundation of Tantra philosophy

The broad, underlying foundation of Tantra philosophy may be summarized briefly as follows:

The universe and everything in it is permeated by a secret energy or power, emanating from the single Source of all being.

This power, although singular in essence, manifests

in three ways, namely, as static inertia, dynamic inertia or mental energy, and as harmonious union of these reacting opposites.

The universe or macrocosm through which these modalities of cosmic force function, is exactly duplicated by the human form as a microcosm.

The Tantrik seeks, therefore, by mystic formularies, rites, and symbols, to identify the corresponding centers of his own body with those of the macrocosm. Ultimately, he seeks union with God Himself.

The importance of the female consort in Tantrik practices stems from the fact that, according to Shastra, every woman is a *shakti;* that is, she embodies the secret, fundamental forces that control the universe.

By correctly joining himself to this line of force, pouring forth from the supreme Absolute, the yogi experiences the ineffable bliss of divine union.

Tantrik scriptures state emphatically that spiritual liberation can come only through experience. States of consciousness cannot be controlled and transcended until and unless they are lived—rapturously, freely, and in all the fullness of their power.

The bond that fetters the soul to *samsara* (created forms) is precisely the dynamic that can deliver it from bondage.

The great mainstream of ancient wisdom

This concept, although brought to its fullest expression by the various Tantrik schools, is not exclusively the fruit of Hindu thought. Actually, many of the basic precepts and rites of Tantrism represent a broad, pre-Indian movement, to which many civilizations have contributed.

In one form or another, for example, the belief that in ritual sexual union, man can elevate and ennoble his life, recurs in all the mystery religions of both East and West.

The student of Tantrism will discover, as he goes along, influences that have entered the currents of Indian thought from the great mainstream of ancient wisdom—esoteric movements from other lands, in which woman incarnates the arcanum of being and becoming.

In strange accord are the devotees of Ishtar in Babylonia; Isis in Egypt; Shing Moo in China; Aphrodite and the Gnostic Sophia in Greece; Diana in Rome; the terrible Kali in India.

In our time, too, perceptive thinkers on both clerical and secular levels, have deeply sensed the power that lies in the union of opposites. To an amazing extent, the "dark moon powers" which the ancients worshipped, have come to permeate modern life.

Several years ago, Winthrop Sargeant, writing in a mass-circulation magazine, observed that 90% of today's movies endlessly repeat the legend of the love goddess.

He points out that there is nothing new about this legend, which has existed in more or less sophisticated forms from remote ages.

"What is new in its twentieth-century American form," he writes, "is its ubiquity and the universal optimism which greets it as a profound religious truth.

"The age-old sex goddess has emerged from the status of a minor folk deity with a rather shady reputation into that of an overwhelming industrialized Molochian idol, to which millions of otherwise sane Americans pay daily tribute." [1]

A prominent Baptist churchman likewise expresses concern over what he terms the cult of the girl in America. Writing in "Christianity and Crisis," he declares:

"Miss America stands in a long line of queens going back to Isis, Ceres and Aphrodite. Everything from the elaborate sexual taboos surrounding her person to the symbolic gifts at her coronation hints at her ancient ancestry. But the real proof comes when we find that the function served by The Girl in our culture is just as much a 'religious' one as that served by Cybele in hers." [2]

The important difference between contemporary attitudes and those of the remote past is that we today have not, by ritual and by self-discipline, turned this creative force into channels of positive spiritual development.

Rather, we have negated and debased it by identifying it only as a "biological function."

So regarded and so misused, it is the potent cup that drinks us downward into spiritual poverty and eventual ruin.

Religion itself must shoulder a large measure of the blame. Not just the Christian religion, but every major faith embraced by mankind. All of them, recognizing sex force as the vital energy of life itself, have sought immediate and absolute control over the sexual mores of humanity. Without exercising such dominion, established religions can not control human adherents.

1 Life Magazine.
2 Harvey Cox: "Cult of The Girl."

Hence the prime importance of sexual taboos in every organized theology.

Certainly, it was Christianity that carried to grotesque extremes the conviction that sex and sin are synonymous.

Taking his cue from the popular ideas of his age and environment, rather than from the example of the Nazarene, the apostle Paul regarded the sexual act as degrading and sinful. Celibacy, he declared, was the ideal state: "I would that all men were even as I."

At the same time, Paul realized the futility of expecting all followers of the New Gospel to forego marriage or to practice chastity within the marital state. Accordingly, "by way of concession, not of commandment," he permitted sexual union within marriage.

The early Church fathers who came after him were less conciliatory. Origen castrated himself to escape sexual desire. Jerome regarded contact with women as corruption, and marriage as the handiwork of Satan. Chrysostom extolled virginity as "greatly superior to marriage." Tertullian boasted of many married converts that they "cancel the debt of their marriage; eunuchs of their own accord, through the desire of the kingdom of heaven."

Coition as a religious rite

This insistence upon suppression of the sex instinct as being favorable to spiritual attainments, runs like a steady refrain through the teachings of saint and theologian alike.

Even in our time, the idea of coition as a religious rite must strike most readers as extraordinary, if not downright blasphemous.

Yet it is the present writer's hope that the thoughts and methodology presented in the following chapters will lead to the discovery that sexual union—with the right partner, at the right time, in the right state of mind—can open the way to a new dimension in life.

After all, say the Tantriks, the universe and everything in it, including man, came into being through the union of the same generative forces—only on a cosmic scale.

Echoing this concept in the West, Havelock Ellis writes that when marriage partners thus approach the conjugal mystery as a sacrament, "they are subtly weaving the invisible cords that bind husband and wife together, more truly and more firmly than the priest of any church.

"And if in the end—as may or may not be—they attain the climax of free and complete union, their human play then has become one with that divine play of creation in which old poets fabled that, out of the dust of the ground and in his own image, some God of Chaos once created Man." [3]

To get the maximum out of this book it is most important that you have the "right" attitude. "Right," as here used means that which is hopeful and affirmative as opposed to "wrong" which is here meant as rejecting and negative. Sexual love is mature love. In our society it may be manifested as distorted love and destructive

[3] Havelock Ellis: "Essays of Love and Virtue."

love, but that is not because of sex but because of a false attitude towards the sexual. When we change our attitude from shameful compulsive indulgence to joyful, choiceful experience, our entire sense of aliveness is liberated and extended.

Too many men and women feel driven to having sexual intercourse with persons whom they seem to dislike and they may repeat the experience with different or the same partners, finding a minimum of pleasure and a maximum sense of inadequacy and frustration. Were such people to merely reverse their basic attitude towards an action they must complete, the action itself would be changed into an experience of joy without shame; of fulfillment without sin or self-degradation. If they were to consider that the sex act was not out of compulsion but out of choice and that the partner was desirable and worthy rather than a pawn in some repulsive, shameful procedure, they would immediately begin to know the experience of being an alive human as compared to an anguished puppet.

It is very possible that the great power of transformation is more in the attitude than anywhere else. As the poets and wise men have said from time immemorial "Love and beauty are in the eyes of the beholder." If we can begin to act (when actions must take place) with the assumption of positive motivation (good), rather than negative compulsion (evil)—then evil is basically defeated. It doesn't have a chance of winning anywhere, especially in sexual love.

Sexual love is beautiful, fulfilling and divine when we rid ourselves of bigoted thinking. Sexual love is the beautiful, hopeful reaching out for the affirmation of living. It is the essence and real purpose of being. We find reflections of such love in the eyes of the child, in the words of the poet, in the world of the artist, in the dreams of the teacher. The power to love is in the subject-self and it is transmitted to the object. Any love which seems to come from an object to a subject is highly questionable.

All through the centuries scholars and scientists pondering the sexual woes of mankind, have believed that were man to know how to prolong the ecstasy which crowns the sexual union, he would discover a greater vision of himself and the universe. He would also conquer many of the sexual frustrations which for thousands of years have limited his growth and sense of self-worth.

Through wholehearted study and application of the sexual principles of Tantra Yoga, man can achieve the sexual potency which enables him to extend the ecstasy crowning sexual union for an hour or more, rather than for the brief seconds he now knows. This is far more than a prolongation, it is the expression of the natural capacity of man and because of this the conclusion of the sexual union does not result in exhaustion or depletion but in complete relaxation and revitalization. This is the goal of Tantra Yoga.

Therefore, in working with this book you should learn to treasure each and every aspect of the sexual union—the touch—the smell—the colors—the sounds—the tastes—the thoughts—the preliminaries—the consummation and the final fulfillment. The more you do this, the greater will be the joys and satisfaction of you and your partner, and your capacity for further renewal.

TANTRA: *The Yoga of Sex*

> "In the beginning, this world was only the Self, in the shape of a person. He looked around; he saw nothing there but himself. First of all, he cried out, "I am!" And then he became frightened; thus one is frightened when alone."
>
> *Brihad-aranyka Upanishad*

1. *The union of opposites*

In attempting to present to the Western reader a clear understanding of Tantrism, we are immediately confronted with a huge semantic obstacle: the word "sex."

No sound symbol in our language is so emotionally charged. None has been given a more limited or narrow meaning.

Until a generation or two ago, the word itself was taboo in public discussion. For it had then, as it has even today, but a single dominant meaning: the biological process of procreation. Something necessary, no doubt, but somehow shameful.

To the Tantrik adept (as to the Western initiate), sex has a vastly more comprehensive and more important meaning.

For them, sex is the cosmic union of opposites, the primordial energy from which arises everything and every being in the universe.

The sacred texts say that during each cycle of cosmic inaction (called the Night of Brahman), there exists but One. It becomes many by an act of will: *"Aham bahu syam—*May I be many."

"He by the power of yoga, became in the act of creation, two-fold; the right half was male and the left was called *prakriti* or female." [1]

The act of generation

In Tantrik ritual, this first act of generation or "shining forth" is symbolized by a grain of gram. And a more appropriate symbol could hardly be found. The gram consists of a partially divided seed, enveloped by a thin sheath or husk. One side of the seed represents the male principle and the other side the female.

At first the seed, although cleft, is of one substance, and joined together in a single body. Then, as generation occurs, the surrounding shell bursts and new life stirs, reaching toward the light.

Such is the bipolar process of creation, from the most microscopic cell to the biggest star.

1 Brahma Vaivartta Purana.

Custodians of the ancient wisdom declare that everything in creation is thus divided into positive and negative, male and female, passive and kinetic, electric and magnetic.

Your own body, for example, is divisible into two halves, each with its own polarity: muscles, limbs, bones, organs of sight and hearing—all come in pairs. Even the brain has two hemispheres. While you have but one heart, it is also divided into right and left sections. The same is true of other internal organs. Structurally, each has two halves, united at a central line.

The feminine or negative side is passive, but magnetic; it attracts to itself, absorbs and stores up potential energy. But bring it into proper contact with the positive or masculine side of nature, and a reaction occurs; power is generated.

The same is true when a predominantly masculine personality is brought into the magnetic "field" of a predominantly feminine one.

"When those two first met," declared a friend, when describing his introduction of a couple who have since become happily married, "you could almost see the sparks fly."

He was, in fact, not far wrong in thus characterizing the kind of discharge that results when the inert potential of *shakti* or the female is fused with the dynamic *Shiva* or the male.

The man and woman referred to experienced the same kind of reaction that makes the "world go 'round" on its axis, crops to grow, or an atomic bomb to explode: reunion of divided poles.

5 ◆ *The union of opposites*

Male-electric, female-magnetic

When such a union between male-electrical and female-magnetic occurs, the couple involved provide a conduit for cosmic force, which flows through them into the earth plane with tremendous power. This power, radiated by them, polarizes the surrounding atmosphere.

Although this phenomenon has been known for centuries in India and Tibet, it was only recently that a Western researcher "discovered" it, independently of any knowledge of Tantrism.

Dr. Rudolph von Urban, a California physician whose practice is largely devoted to marital problems and sexology, said the manifestation was first reported to him by an Oriental patient.

The patient, also a doctor of medicine, told Dr. von Urban that the curious incident had occurred during the first week of his marriage to a beautiful Syrian girl. He said his wife and he lay together on a couch, naked and in close contact for about an hour, caressing each other, but not consummating the union. The room was in total darkness (a condition, incidentally, that is strictly forbidden in Tantrik ritual).

When the couple separated and stood up, the young physician was amazed to see that his wife was surrounded by a corona of greenish-blue, mystic light.

Slowly, the husband reached out his hand toward his bride. When his open palm was within an inch of her breast, an electric spark, painful to both, crackled between them.

"We both shrank back," he recounted.

With this strange case as a point of departure, Dr. von Urban later conducted a carefully controlled study of the phenomenon. The resulting data provided material for an excellent book, based on "the conviction that differences in bio-electrical potential exist in male and female bodies, and that an exchange between these two types of electricity takes place in proper sex union." [2]

Cosmic forces

The Tantrik texts leave no doubt as to the importance and the dangers inherent in such a union as that described. The powerful cosmic forces that surround us at all times, seeking expression through polarization, can vastly alter our whole lives.

Properly understood and used, such a union can intensify and expand the knowledge, talents and mental powers of both partners. The singer will sing as never before, the poet find a greater release into the world of creative imagination; the mathematician will experience less difficulty in arriving at solutions to the most difficult problems.

Here, in fact, is the secret knowledge underlying all Tantrik procedure. It is the basic power that attracts or repels other people. It can bestow health or cause disease. It can be used to obtain wealth, to unlock the mysteries of the unconscious. Ultimately, it can bring the *sadhaka* (aspirant) to the final goal of all yoga—that of spiritual perfection.

2 Rudolph von Urban, M.D.: "Sex Perfection and Marital Happiness."

Weird practices of
"Brothers of the Left Hand"

In many parts of Tibet, Tantrik magicians, so-called "brothers of the left-hand," have evolved powerful and frightening ways of using the energy derived from sexual union—not always to good ends.

One order of Tibetan nuns is known to keep spies among the general populace for the purpose of locating and enspelling sexually vigorous young men. These victims are then taken to remote convents where they are held in thrall and used as a source of psychic galvanism for various occult practices.

If we are to believe the account of an English writer, women are similarly spirited away by the Dugpas—a sect of Red Cap lamas—for the same purposes.[3]

Another and even more dangerous kind of vampirism is secretly practiced in some parts of India. A young and healthy person of the opposite sex is chosen for this technique. Knowing that sublimated sexual energy is stored in the spinal fluid in a form known as ojas, the Tantrik of the left-hand inserts a hollow needle into the donor's spinal column between the vertebrae and near the base, withdrawing a small amount of fluid.

Then, in a similar operation, he takes from his own spinal column a smaller amount of the fluid. The two are mixed together and re-injected into his own spine.

It must be strongly emphasized that this procedure is extremely dangerous and should never be undertaken by the layman. It and other practices mentioned in the foregoing paragraphs, are cited merely to indicate to the

[3] Elizabeth Sharpe: "Secrets of the Kaula Circle."

reader the wide scope of Tantrism. At one end of the spectrum, we have the loftiest motives and noblest ideals. At the other, we find negative sensuality, vampirism and magic.

Qualifications for safe and successful results

Both aspects of Tantra, however, have one thing in common. Both make use of the same primal energy which, like any force of nature, may be put to good or evil use, depending upon the character of the user.

As a matter of fact, most Tantrik texts carefully spell out the qualifications necessary for the safe and successful practice of *sandhana*. They specifically exclude the voluptuary, the drunkard, the lewd person, the glutton, and the lecher.

In the West, sexual intercourse is defined as the act of copulation, or at best, the act together with the love play, if any, preceding it.

The Vedic scriptures, on the other hand, view all relations between persons of opposite sex as varying degrees of coition.

Even contemplating or visualizing the act will, to some extent, change the thinker's polarity and is, therefore, to be regarded as one kind of sex act.

In this connection, the words of Jesus seem to indicate a similar view, for he declared:

"But I say unto you, That whosoever looketh on a woman to lust after her hath committed adultery with her already in his heart." [4]

4 Matthew V:28.

Eight aspects of sexual intercourse

In the Hindu texts, sexual intercourse is said to have eight aspects. These are enumerated as: (1) *smarnanam* or allowing the thoughts to dwell upon it; (2) *kirtanam* or discussing it with another; (3) *keli*—keeping company with the opposite sex; (4) *prekshenam* or flirting; (5) *guhyabhashanam* or intimate conversation with a person of the opposite sex; (6) *samkalpa* or the desire for coition; (7) *adhyavasayam* or firm determination to indulge; and (8) *kriyanishpatti* or physical copulation.

Thus, many who believe themselves sexually chaste are, in fact, only sexually subtle. Their conduct differs from that of the debauchee, not in kind, but merely in degree.

Eventually, the Freudians notwithstanding, there will dawn the realization that the libido, manifesting as sexual desire, is not lust per se, but the yearning for completion.

It is the ultimate destiny of the soul to achieve that completion through the union of polar opposites within his own body. Thus reborn as the divine androgyne—the offspring of Shiva and Shakti—the soul will then inhabit only the higher *lokas* or planes of existence.

Is not such a teleology implied also in the Christian scripture in which Jesus says:

"For in the resurrection they neither marry, nor are given in marriage, but are as the angels of God in heaven." [5]

[5] Matthew XXII:30.

Levels of being

Even in our present state, each of us may function as a man on one level of being and as a woman on another.

According to Tantra Shastra, while each of us is predominantly male or female in the physical world, that polarity does not remain the same in the other six *lokas* or zones of existence.

If you are a woman, for example, on the mental plane you probably are oriented to the masculine pole, and mentally function as a man. A man's mind, on the other hand, is usually feminine in character.

But in the subtle interplay of forces that characterize our invisible relationships, it is the degree of intensity that determines polarity—or if you prefer, sex.

In any man-woman relationship, the partner expressing the stronger qualities of a given plane will be male on that plane, irrespective of his or her sex in the physical body.

This means, of course, that a woman may be feminine, absorbing, magnetic in her relationship to one man; but positive, masculine and dominant in her rapport with another. The same is true of a man in his relations with different women.

Herein lies a valuable clue to be used in diagnosing many conflicts and inharmonies of modern marriages.

It may also provide a means of understanding and resolving many discords within ourselves. For each of us exists and functions on more than one plane or level of consciousness. Each of these levels has its own polarity, depending upon the intensity of our feeling in that dimension.

The ancient wisdom of the Tantras asserts that man's

subtle "bodies" or spiritual modalities, polarize each other on a descending scale. The more highly-evolved level of consciousness is always dominant and masculine in its relation to the one just below it.

Conversely, the denser body will be feminine-negative in its relation to the higher.

This line of authority, so to speak, or regulation from above, is tremendously important to the understanding and practice of Tantra Yoga, as will become evident in what follows.

"What is here is elsewhere.
What is not here is nowhere."
—*Vishvasara Tantra.*

2. *Secrets of breath control*

Anyone even slightly familiar with the practice of yoga in any of its numerous forms, knows that the spinal column has a vital place in the yogic scheme of things.

Almost without exception, books on the subject show the reader in detail, either by means of illustrations or textual description, the structure of the spinal cord and its occult centers, called *chakras*.

But, beyond a brief account of the spiritual physiology involved and an admonition always to keep the spine erect while engaged in breathing exercises, little more is offered.

For the Tantrik *sadhaka,* on the other hand, the spinal column is of prime importance. This is because it is literally the central axis of his being.

"The Staff of Meru"

Tantrik doctrine teaches that man's vertebral column corresponds to a hollow stone core running through the center of our planet, constituting the earth's axis. Hindu mythology describes a mountain called Meru, situated somewhere in the depressed area of the north polar region. It is traditionally the dwelling place of the Asura giants, and playground of the Vedic gods.

Because man's cerebro-spinal axis is considered to be analogous to the earth's pole, in Tantrik literature it is referred to as Mt. Meru, or as Meru-danda ("the staff of Meru").

According to the *Agamas,* every man is a universe. Each of our bodies is a microcosm, embodying all the individual forms of life and geographical configurations of creation, from the lowest to the highest.

As earth scientists venture forth to explore other planets and distant worlds, they will find, in essence, only what is upon earth and within man. So teach the Tantrik Shastras. Hence the statement in the Vishva-sara Tantra: "What is here is elsewhere. What is not here is nowhere."

Such a concept will at once appear absurd to those familiar only with Western physiology and science, which deals only with the physical body and gross matter.

But for the occultist, accustomed to peering into the invisible side of nature, there is nothing new in the idea of these correspondences. Hermetic and Cabbalistic philosophers long since have declared:

"As above, so below."

The five regions of the vertebral axis

Coming to the question of most immediate concern, that of the human body, Tantrik literature describes the vertebral axis as being divided into five parts or "regions."

Starting upward from the lowest, the coccygeal (which consists of the first four incomplete vertebrae), the sections include the sacral region (five vertebrae), the dorsal or back (twelve vertebrae); and the cervical or neck (seven vertebrae).

Each of these regions or zones, upon careful examination will be found to exhibit different characteristics in the overall function of the central nervous system.

It is important for the student to bear these divisions in mind, since they are areas of the physical body whose locations roughly correspond with the vital centers of radiation in the subtle body, with which we shall presently be concerned.

In its physical structure, the spine consists of a series of thirty-three vertebrae, placed one upon the other, to form a bony pediment. In addition to providing a support for the head and torso, the column forms a hollow, protective passage for the spinal cord.

The cord extends downward from the fourth ventricle of the brain to the coccygeal region, where it narrows to a thin, hair-like ending called the *filum terminale.*

In keeping with the binary nature of created structures, previously mentioned, the cord is formed of two symmetrical halves joined together along a central line. In this instance, the line of juncture is really a minute conduit called the *canalis centralis* or central canal.

This tiny, central canal is of prime concern to the Tantrik *sadhaka,* for it is through this passage that he raises the sleeping mystic force called *kundalini,* from the base of the spine to the head. As it rises, it vitalizes six centers of power along its invisible course to the brain.

In the Hindu lexicon, the channel is called the *sushumna.* Some Tantrik writings also mention two other and even smaller channels for psychic energy, unknown to Western anatomy. These are called the *vajrini* and the *chitrini.*

The *vajrini* is the larger of the two, and carries inside its walls the *chitrini.* The latter is described as "fine as a spider's web."

Both these occult tubules are perceptible only to psychic vision. Indeed, the entire occult anatomy, as set forth in the *Agamas,* is invisible to routine procedures of dissection. No doubt it is for this reason, and because the astral structures disappear from the gross physical body at the time of death, that Western science denies their existence.

"Door of Brahma"

An opening at the lower end of the *chitrini* channel is often referred to by Tantriks as the Door of Brahma, because through it must pass the psychic current that will bring cosmic consciousness to the yogi.

Outside the *sushumna* canal, and on the right and left side of it, respectively, are two other important conduits called the *pingala* and the *ida*.

They coil upward around the *sushumna*, forming "knots" at the points where they intersect along the spine.

The *pingala* passage starts from the left testicle of the male (left ovary of the female), and ends at the right nostril. The *ida* originates at the right testicle (or ovary), and terminates at the left nostril.

At a point between the eyebrows, the two mystical "arteries" unite with the *sushumna*, weaving at that site a threefold "knot," known as the Third Eye.

For the Tantrik, our gross body and its interpenetrating psychic bodies are constantly energized by various currents of life force, which determine the function and state of health of our physical being.

This primal energy, known as *prana*, operates freely through the *ida*, *pingala*, and the *sushumna*.

Alternating breath flow

Let us consider first the act of breathing. Although it is nowhere noted in the literature of Western medicine, the breath does not flow equally through both nostrils, except for very brief intervals during the day.

Instead, it will normally issue from the left nostril for an interval of perhaps twenty-four minutes, then shift to the right nostril for a like period of time.

The two astral ducts—*pingala* and *ida*—convey cosmic energy to the nostrils.

The current which flows from the right nostril is masculine, electrical, hot, of a fiery red color to psychic vision. Being a polarization of the solar principle of creation, it is commonly called by yogis the "sun breath."

The vital air which flows through the *ida* and left nostril is feminine, magnetic, cool and pale white to astral vision. Being of the lunar principle of creation, it is known as the "moon breath." It is the nourisher of the physical body.

When the breath flow is through both nostrils simultaneously, it is said that the combined energies of sun, moon and fire enter the *sushumna* canal. It is then that the yogi achieves psychic powers, makes time stand still, and possesses knowledge of the future.

But for those not versed in yoga, the brief interval in which the breath flows equally from both nostrils is extremely perilous. It is during this interim that accidents and death occur, losses take place, and failures are likely.

Among the Tantriks in both India and Tibet, it is considered dangerous to leave a place where both sun and moon breaths are flowing. It is not uncommon to see those who cannot change the breath flow at will, resort to one or another of the physical means of changing the flow, usually to the left nostril.

A Kaul once told me that any curse uttered during the

time that *prana* was moving in the *sushumna* canal, would almost certainly come to pass. He believed it was this terrible power that witches of the Middle Ages used to bring sickness and grief to their victims.

En passant, it is interesting to note that several Theosophical and Western texts state that the Caduceus or winged staff of Mercury is a diagrammatic representation of the invisible cerebro-spinal axis. The rod itself, of course, represents the spine. The two serpents that entwine the staff are identified with the right and left channels, *pingala* and *ida.* The small sphere at the top of the rod represents the pineal gland; and the "wings of Mercury" are the flames emitted when the fiery *kundalini* or psychic current rises inside the spinal canal to contact the final center of power (the *sahasrara*).

Sun and Moon breath

But let us return to further consideration of the alternating breath flow. The doctors of Hindu Tantrism have set forth in great detail the significance of both the position taken by the breath flow through the nostrils, and the distance the exhalation extends from the nostrils.

It may be taken as a general rule that the moon breath (through the left nostril) affects the sympathetic nervous system. It represents the influx of Shakti or mother principle and as such, both nourishes and regulates body functions. It is also the source of desire, dreams, wisdom, fantasies, and all the "dark moon powers" of woman.

The sun breath (through the right nostril) nurtures

and sustains the vasomotor system. It is the source of action, violence, body heat, lust, and all the virile pursuits of the warrior.

The *sushumna* breath (through both nostrils simultaneously) controls man's destiny, death, and time. Many yogis claim to have prolonged their lifespan by taking *prana* (the cosmic, primordial energy behind breath) through the *sushumna* canal to the vital center in the brain and holding it there.

The kind of breath flow of the parents during intercourse will even determine the sex of the child, if conception occurs.

Thus, if the man's breath is through the *pingala* or right side, and the woman's through the *ida* or left nostril, the resulting child will be male, according to Tantrik doctrine.

Conversely, if the man's breath flow is through the *ida* and the woman's through the *pingala,* the child will be a girl.

If, on the other hand, both parents are in the same breath (whether *pingala* or *ida*), the child will have a predisposition to homosexuality.

In addition to determining simply whether his breath flow is through the right or left nostril, the Tantrik *sadhaka* also seeks to ascertain which of the five elements —water, air, fire, earth and ether—rules the breath at a given moment.

This is done by learning to judge the exact way in which the breath is passing from the nostril.

When the flow is precisely through the center of the nostril, for example, it is an "earth breath."

When it passes across the lower peripheral portion of the nostril as it flows in and out, it is a "water breath."

If the breath, when vigorously inhaled or exhaled, touches the upper wall inside the nostril, it is moving with the element fire.

It is an "air breath" when the flow passes down the left side of the nasal wall.

If the flow touches the right wall of the nostril, it is an "ether breath."

Actions, thoughts, decision, and so on, which occur during the time the breath is in an earth cycle will have positive or fortunate results.

During the ether and the airy cycles, on the other hand, actions or ideas end in loss, destruction, death.

The fire element in the breath also brings grief, fear, changes, fevers, defeats.

Yogis versed in Tantrism say that if you ask a seer regarding the future success of some undertaking when the breath flow is in the earth element, you will realize a positive or fortunate outcome. Per contra, if a "fire breath" or an "air breath" should prevail at the time of such a query, a negative answer is in order, and failure can almost certainly be predicted.

Tantrik opinion also holds that each elemental breath has its own characteristic vibratory rate or color; its own shape, and its own distance of projection from the nostrils.

Earth breath is yellow and square; it extends from the nares three inches.

Water breath is white and circular; it projects from the nostril twelve inches.

Fire breath is red and triangular; its trajectory is four inches in length.

Air breath is green and in the form of an oblique line: it flows outward a distance of eight inches.

Of the *akasha* or ether breath nothing definite is known. It is believed by some Tantrik authorities to be without special color or form. It is the vital cosmic air that is the all-pervading rhythm of the universe.

Orthodox Shakta doctrine states that the *ida* or the *pingala* will flow more powerfully on certain days of the week. *Ida* is strongest on Wednesday, Thursday, Friday and Sunday; and it is especially puissant on the days during the light of the moon.

Pingala or right nostril flow is more potent on Monday, Tuesday, and Saturday; this is true especially during the dark half of the lunar cycle.

The great importance assigned to the course of the breath flow in determining the successful outcome of given activities is based upon a fundamental yogic postulate. It is that the flow of air in the gross body is linked with a corresponding current of *prana* or psychic energy in the subtle or astral body. The two function more or less in parallel, and can mutually influence each other.

Human activities to be undertaken

Shakta literature enumerates in some detail the kind of human activities to be undertaken during the sun breath and the moon breath, respectively.

The lists include an almost endless tally of actions and ideas, but the following are a good cross-section:

While the breath is flowing through the *pingala* (right nostril), one should undertake:

Generally, all actions involving physical exertion, passion, force, crime, or combat.

The enticement of women (if you are a man). Embracing, caressing, sexual intercourse.

All forms of active sport such as swimming, hunting, riding, and so on.

Inflicting punishment upon others, or causing them pain.

Selling anything.

Seizing anything by stealth and/or by theft.

Entering into a contest or debate of any kind.

Gambling and cheating.

Using weapons correctly, accurately, and safely.

Partaking of food and drink.

Taking a bath.

Exorcising ghosts or practicing any occult art.

When the breath flow is through the *ida* or left nostril, it is a propitious time to perform the following:

Generally, all activities of a calm, gentle, steady nature.

Practicing any of the arts—painting, singing, writing, composing, and so on.

Buying anything.

Studying music or dancing.

Beginning a course of study in any subject.

Going to church, or joining in services of worship.

Study of science.

Planting or sowing seeds.

Earning a livelihood.

Engaging in any business transaction.

Preparing food for any purpose.

Taking part in wedding ceremonies.

Travel from one place to another, especially if it is a long journey.

Visiting with friends or relatives.

Speaking with persons in authority on any topic.

Upon entering a house, especially one not your own.

The Tantrik canon also mentions a number of situations deliberately brought about by the yogi's breath control.

For example, it is said that if a man, being in the sun-breath, draws into his right nostril the breath from a woman's left nostril, she will give him lasting love and devotion. This is particularly true if the breath exchange occurs during a close embrace or sexual intercourse.

A man should seek to win a woman's favor at the moment when the breath flow is changing over from the right nostril to the left. For a woman, of course, just the reverse would be true.

Since the manner in which the vital energy (behind the breath) thus determines the course of our lives, it is important to know how to change the breath flow as desired.

How to control the "breath flow"

There are advanced *sadhakas* who can change the breath simply by an act of will. For the majority who can not, however, several techniques have been developed for accomplishing the same purpose.

Perhaps the easiest method for the Western student is to lie down on the side opposite from that through which he wishes the breath to flow. Thus, if you wish the breath to flow through the right nostril, lie on your left side, and vice versa. You will soon be able to perceive the exact moment when the change-over from one nostril to the other occurs. Normally, it will not take more than two or three minutes. If you have a cold or nasal congestion from some other cause, a little more time may be required.

One way of hastening the change when using this method, is to prop yourself on your elbow, supporting your head with your hand, your thumb resting firmly under the ear, and the fingers pressed against the forehead.

Pressure in and around the arm-pit of the side opposite the desired flow will also initiate a change-over. To avoid attracting attention when this method is used in the presence of others, it may be effected by dropping your arm over the back of a chair. In India and parts of Tibet, it is a common sight to see yogis equipped with short T-shaped staffs (called hangsa danda) upon which they lean for this purpose.

Another means of correcting or changing the breath flow is to sit upon the floor and draw the right or left knee, as desired, up to the arm-pit and lean heavily upon it.

Yet another procedure, which calls for no extraordinary prowess on the part of the shakti student is to massage the ankle and great toe, again opposite the side through which you wish the breath to flow.

Quite aside from using the great toe as a means for changing the breath flow, Tantrik aspirants are taught to massage this toe (on both feet) regularly. They are told that a nerve terminating in the large toe regulates all cyclic changes and rhythms in the entire body.

A final and quite obvious way to cause the breath to

flow through a given nostril is to plug the opposite one. When this is done, a piece of clean cotton cloth is rolled into a kind of small ball and inserted into the nostril.

If not wilfully changed by the *sadakha,* the breath flow will continue to alternate back and forth, changing from one nostril to the other.

However, most gurus strongly counsel their students to practice *swara sadhana*—that is, to make the breath flow solely through the left nostril from sunrise to sunset; and through the right nostril from sunset to sunrise. Faithful performance of this procedure, they insist, will ward off disease, prolong the lifespan of the yogi, and confer wisdom.

After a little experimenting with the techniques described, you will soon be able to control the breath flow, directing it through the right or left nostril as you desire.

It is well to undertake this simple and easy exercise at once. A mastery of breath flow (that is, of the pranic airs) constitutes an operational constant in all the Tantrik practices which follow.

"Man's consciousness has no fixed boundary."
—Avalon: Shakti & Shakta

3. *Wheels of ecstasy*

In this our age of fear, anxiety and materialism, the doctrine of Tantra yoga reminds us of a long-forgotten truth:

We are in continual, direct touch with an order of existence far higher than that of earth.

In the profound depths of our being, we receive guidance from the mind of God; we commune with saints; we walk the ancient paths of mystery beyond time and space, to the remotest star.

Entities unseen, both good and bad, monstrous and beautiful surround us and interpenetrate us and live within the gross body we identify as ourselves.

Tantrik preceptors, like mystics of all countries and all epochs, not only take note of these beings, but seek to gain spiritual insight from them if they are of higher worlds; or to command them if they are of the lower orders.

To the Western student, steeped as he is in the traditions of empirical knowledge, such a belief may appear to be a metaphysical presumption, or at best, a wholly subjective experience, valid only for the person for whom it occurs.

If such modes of cognition are real, where is the mechanism that makes them possible? (For in our time, even the function of the brain is believed to be that of a servo-mechanism, or a highly sophisticated computer.)

Your causal body and your subtle body

The Tantriks answer quite simply that there is more to the human being than meets the eye or that can be measured and analyzed in laboratory procedures.

In fact, they might add, there is only about one third of you in evidence. The rest is invisible.

That is merely another way of saying that, in addition to your gross physical body made up of dense matter, you have two other bodies.

These are called by various names, the most common being the causal body and the subtle body.

According to Shakta doctrine, the causal body is the most enduring of the three. It was the original luminous consciousness out of which the subtle and physical bodies evolved. It is, so to speak, the immediate envelope or sheath of the soul (*Jivatma*), which lasts until final liberation from our round of deaths and rebirths.

Yogis say that during states of dreamless sleep, the causal body provides a point of direct interchange of psychic energy between the two lower bodies and the cosmic sphere.

The subtle body has been identified with the so-called unconscious or the subconscious mind. Involuntary functions of the physical body, including heart-beat, breathing, digestion, excretion, and endocrine secretion, are controlled by the subtle body, which operates continuously. It is without volition, and responds to suggestions and commands from any source: words, sounds, odors, colors, size, and so on.

The psychic currents that pass from one body to another do so by means of invisible conduits called *nadis,* woven throughout the subtle body "like threads in a spider web." Hence the name Tantra, which means "a web."

It must be understood that while these minute ducts sometimes parallel in their courses, nerves and veins of the physical body, they should not be identified with either.

They are, rather, etheric vessels whose function is to convey streams of polarized energy throughout the gross body as well as the subtle body. Being part of the spiritual anatomy, they are invisible to physical sight.

There is a vast number of these *nadis,* of different sizes, spreading throughout the body. Authorities are divided on the question of the exact number. Some say 350,000; others 200,000; and yet others, 80,000. The largest body of opinion, however, agrees on 72,000 as the correct number.

All the *nadis* have their point of origin in an important center of the subtle body, called the *kanda*. The texts describe it as an egg-shaped bulb, covered with a membrane. The *kanda* is situated in the physical body at a point midway between the anus and genitals. Some texts say approximately nine finger-breadths above the reproductive organs and twelve above the anus.

The vital currents which these psychic channels carry to nourish our bodies, are fed to the physical organism through focal centers called *chakras*.

In Sanskrit, the word *chakra* means wheel or disc. Since the subtle centers appear to psychic sight to be round, vibrating vortices, it is easy to see why the word "wheel" was used to describe them.

Many writings also refer to them as lotuses because, at times, they may resemble that flower, with a given number of "petals."

The *chakras* are six in number, each with its individual colors and number of "spokes" or "petals." Each spoke vibrates at the rate of one of the fifty root sounds of creation, represented in the literature by a corresponding letter of the Sanskrit alphabet.

Like the *nadis* or mystical veins, the *chakras* are part of your invisible anatomy. They are, however, correlated with the endocrine system of the gross body. For that reason and because there is a mutual influence between the visible and invisible bodies, a number of texts on yoga have incorrectly identified the subtle ganglia (chakras) with the physical glands. For example, a Hindu physician, recently referred to the centers as "neurohormonal mechanisms." [1]

1 Rammurti Mishra, M.D.: "Fundamentals of Yoga."

It is true that the currents of life force or vital airs as they are sometimes called, flow most vigorously when the physical organs and the etheric structures that inter-penetrate them are both functioning harmoniously.

The flow of vitalizing energy from the cosmic sphere can be greatly reduced and enfeebled by illness or abuses of the physical body.

For example, irregular or wrong breathing, impure air, excessive use of alcohol, and so on, can result in serious disturbances within your subtle bodies. These disturbances, in turn, are reflected in the physical body in what medicine today knows as psychosomatic illness.

Seven vital centers of radiation

Let us take a closer look at these vital centers of radiation. For, without at least an elementary knowledge of them, and of how to stimulate their activity, the practice of yoga is merely an intellectual exercise.

MULADHARA

The first and lowest in the six wheels or centers is called the *muladhara*. It is situated at the base of the spinal column, about midway between the anal orifice and the genital organs. Four red petals (*nadis*) emanate from it.

In the center of the *chakra* is a yellow square, which is the earth element. Within the square appears an inverted triangle that encloses the mysterious psychic energy called *kundalini*. This energy is often called "serpent power" because in its quiescent form, it lies coiled around the base of the spinal column. Tantrik texts describe *kundalini* as "luminous as lightning, shining in the hollow of this lotus like a chain of brilliant lights."

The *muladhara* energy is the electrical force of creation. It is the cohesive power of matter, the so-called atomic glue of science. In man, it governs the sense of smell and stimulates our knowledge of speech.

According to Tantrik doctrine, meditation upon this center leads to the mastery of desire, envy, anger, and passion. It is the etheric analogue of the gonads in the physical body.

SVADISTHANA

As we proceed upward along the central spinal canal (*sushumna*), the second center of radiation is the one called *svadisthana*.

Situated at the root of the genitals, it has six vermilion *nadis* emanating from it. The texts describe a white crescent moon, mystically related to the element water, in the center of the *chakra*.

In man, the center governs the sense of taste, and controls the function of the kidneys and lower abdominal region of the physical body, including the legs.

By meditation upon this center, the yogi acquires the "dark moon powers," among them the ability to see and to communicate with entities who inhabit the astral worlds.

In India and Tibet, it is said that one about to travel on water or who is threatened with floods, must seek mastery over the situation by stimulating this center.

It is analogous to, and influences, the adrenal glands.

MANIPURA

Continuing our ascent of Mt. Meru, or the spinal column, the next center of force we encounter is the *manipura.*

It is commonly known as the "navel lotus" because it is situated in the lumbar region, opposite the navel.

Its vibratory rate makes it appear to clairvoyant vision as "the color of heavy-laden rain clouds." According to a description given in the Satchakra Nirupana, a bright orange-red triangle is seen at the center, on three sides of which are swastikas. Ten *nadis* emanate from it. It is related to the element fire.

Psychic currents from the *manipura* flow into the internal organs of the physical body in the epigastric region, thereby controlling the stomach, liver, intestines, and so on. The center is also related to the menstrual flow in women, and influences the eyesight in both sexes.

Those versed in the Tantras say that the *manipura chakra* is of great importance in the practice of magic and alchemy. A knowledge and mastery of the plexus frees the yogi from all disease, fulfills secret desires, and enables him to penetrate the deepest consciousness of other minds.

It is by stimulation of this *chakra* that the fire-walkers

of India are able to walk upon glowing coals with impunity. One text, the Gheranda Samhita, goes even further. It states flatly that the *sadhaka* who knows how to enter the "seed of fire" in the pericarp of this lotus, can be thrown into the midst of a roaring blaze (as the Biblical trio—Meshach, Shadrach and Abednego—were cast into the fiery furnace) and "remain alive without fear of death."

The center is also used in discovering the location of hidden treasure.

Its physical point of focus in the physical body is the pancreas.

Each of us has stored in the solar plexus an amazing reservoir of psychic power, and we shall have occasion to use some of it in one of the exercises to be explained later on in this book.

ANAHATA

The fourth center of force is the *anahata,* situated in the chest. It is often called the heart lotus because it is the heart and cardiac region of the physical body. Deep red in color, it has twelve mystic ducts emanating from it.

In the middle of the *anahata* are two intersecting triangles (known to the Kabala as the Seal of Solomon, symbolizing the macro- and microcosm). Within these triangles is the core of our individual being, the very spark of the divine, which glows "like the steady tapering flame of a lamp."

To meditate upon this center is to practice yoga in

one of its highest forms, for within it will be heard the Shabda Brahma, the primordial, mystical syllable Om, which is the combined sound of the universe, the tone of all creation. There are many varieties of this sound, the most common being the following: the sound of a swarm of bees; a waterfall; humming, like that of telephone wires; roaring of the sea; ringing of a bell; rustling of tiny silver chains; flute notes; shrill, high whistling; the sound of a drum; distant thunder.

The *anahata* embodies the element air. It governs the sense of touch, the penis, the circulatory system and the locomotor system.

Extravagant claims of paranormal powers are made by some yogis who have concentrated upon this center in their practices. These powers include hearing and seeing at great distances; becoming invisible; precognition; and even the ability to enter and take over another person's body.

It should be emphasized here that the acquiring of such powers, if indeed that is possible, lies quite outside the scope of exercises included in the present work.

Most aspirants will feel amply rewarded if results promised by the more practical *agamas* are forthcoming. The latter state merely that the practitioner of Tantrik doctrine will be beloved of Lakshmi—that is, that material fortune will smile on him.

"His inspired speech flows like a stream of water." [2]

He will be attractive to the opposite sex and eventually will be the recipient of cosmic love. "Having enjoyed in this world the best of pleasure, he in the end goes to the abode of Liberation." [3]

2 Satchakra Nuripana: Woodroffe trans.
3 Kalikarana: Commentary.

The *anahata* influences the function of the thymus gland in the gross body.

VISHUDDHA

Ascending the subtle channel inside the spinal column, the next point at which the invisible world meets the visible is the *vishuddha* or "Great Purity" center.

As the name suggests, this plexus is associated with a highly developed order of being. It is the doorway to the plane of eternal wisdom.

Its location is the base of the throat. It has sixteen subtle "spokes" of smoky purple, which spread through the laryngeal and pharyngeal regions at the junction of the spinal column and the medulla oblongata.

Tantrik opinion asserts that the center of the *vishuddha* glows brilliantly when the yogi is spiritually advanced.

The *chakram* is described as "the region of ether, circular and white like the full moon." [4]

It controls the sense of hearing, the skin, the mouth, and the respiration.

"Whoever will concentrate upon this center becomes a sage in the sacred knowledge, a prince among yogis." [5]

The exoteric organ related to the *vishuddha* is the thyroid gland.

4 Satchakra Nirupana: v. 28, 29.
5 Shiva Samhita: v. 5.

AJNA

The *ajna* is situated between the eyebrows at the site polarized as that of "the Third Eye." It is known as the center of command.

It is "beautifully white, like the winter moon," and has two subtle channels or "spokes" emanating from it. In diagram, the center, with its two wing-like *nadis* atop the staff of Meru, suggests the wand of Mercury, which may be a symbol of the same esoteric truth.

The center of command is, appropriately enough, the seat of man's mental faculties. It is the abode of the individual consciousness, but also a meeting place with the divine; for at this center the aspirant may hear the voice of his spiritual guru and be initiated into the secret knowledge of Tantra.

Meditation upon the *ajna* will result in the *sadhaka's* being released from the consequences of actions in previous incarnations.

"The yogi who meditates upon this center at the moment of his death, when the breath is leaving his body, dissolves into and becomes one with the Supreme Being." [6]

In the physical body, the pituitary gland is correlated with the *ajna*.

SAHASRARA

Above the *ajna* lies the "thousand-petalled lotus" called the *sahasrara,* where the three principal arteries of the subtle body come together.

[6] Shiva Samhita: v. 5.

Here, the final goal of the Tantrik aspirant is achieved: the union of the opposite polarities, the wedding of Shiva and Shakti; male and female; electric and magnetic; solar and lunar.

Since this final and greatly augmented plexus is above and beyond the earth plane, most Tantrik writers do not designate it a *chakram* at all, but consider it a transcendental point of focus, where the soul enters and leaves the physical body at time of birth and death.

The site in the physical body nearest to the *sahasrara* is the crown of the head, where the slightly depressed area corresponds to the polar region of our globe.

As suggested earlier, the line of authority or regulation of our bodies, is always from the higher or more subtle, downward to the lower and more dense. Consequently, the *sahasrara* controls the six centers below it.

In various individuals, the area of the center's expansion differs. In persons who are not greatly advanced spiritually, the vibratory rays are pale and condensed at the top of the head. In the more highly developed, the prismatic colors of the "petals" cover the head like a cap of glowing jewels.

By meditation upon this center, the yogi acquires strange powers and conquers the twin enemies: time and death.

4. *The true beginning*

The serious student may well ask at this point:

Is there a prescribed order or program in Tantrik practice? If so, what is the first step?

The answer to such a query is that there is a definite procedure to be followed.

But before considering in detail the preliminary exercises in the *disciplina arcani,* let us re-examine for a moment the underlying theory of Shaktism.

The thing which immediately distinguishes it from other forms of yoga is that, whereas other schools teach techniques aimed at self-denial and the extinction of sensuous experience, Tantra urges the fullest possible involvement in life.

As Sir John Woodroffe wrote of the *sadakha,* "he attains liberation, eating the sweet fruits of the world." [1]

Such a doctrine should not, however, be mistaken for hedonism.

*"He who realizes the truth of the body
can then come to know the
truth of the universe."*

Tantrism is a goal-directed course of action. The end in view, as previously stated, is the union of the two polar streams of life force—a reintegration that produces spiritual illumination.

Live life and live it more fully, is the admonition of the Shakta canon. Plunge into being with sharpened awareness.

The world is indeed a wedding. In every act of every day, you are either the bridegroom or the bride. You are the strong or the weak, the electric or the magnetic, the lover or the beloved.

And from these marriages, these fecundating unions, comes the renewal of life. By the act of procreation— whether it be physical, mental or spiritual—you are to a degree reborn. Man was born to change. Only thereby can he grow and attain freedom.

In short, for a man attuned to his soul, each rebirth

1 Sir John Woodroffe: "Principles of Tantra."

is into a new world of thought and feeling—one of greater reality, greater response to being.

For Tantrism holds that the world is not an illusion, but real. Real flesh experience is the extension of the soul's purpose. Only in our deeper feelings, only in love, is the divine creative force registered, not in intellection.

Truth therefore, can not be taught; it can only be lived.

It is man's way to teach. It is God's way to experience. Teachings are but the substance of other men's experience, other men's thoughts, fossilized into permanent beliefs or creeds. They are but tradition made law.

That is the meaning of the passage in the Ratnasara which declares that "he who realizes the truth of the body can then come to know the truth of the universe."

For that reason, the practice of Tantra yoga starts with the body and its functions. That is the true beginning.

The first objective is to cleanse the principal *nadis* or astral channels previously described, so that psychic currents may unite and flow through them from the subtle body into the physical body.

Cleansing is achieved by regulation of the breath, a technique known as pranayama. As the term itself implies, the procedure is really aimed at a control of *prana*. This fact calls for a further explanation. What is *prana*?

Essentially, *prana* is nothing more than cosmic energy. It is the sum total of all primal force in the universe, whether in an inert, transitional or in a dynamic state.

It is the tremendous power released from the atom when it is fissioned or fused. It is the unseen, ever-present reality behind all movement, all thinking, willing, doing.

For biological organisms, including man, the most important gross manifestation of *prana* is breathing. For in the act of breathing, according to the Shastras, we absorb not only oxygen, but also the basic life-force— *prana.*

When breathing ceases, the body's polarity undergoes radical change: the positive, electrical forces of the body, in the form of acid, flood into the negative, alkaline of the blood. The body's mechanism becomes static, ceasing to function. The once-living organism ceases breathing and dies.

It follows that Tantriks, in common with all yogis, attach considerable importance to regulating the breath.

Control the breath, they say, and you can clear the subtle passages of the etheric body and direct life currents through them. In the gross body, the central nervous system is purified and vitalized. Digestion is accelerated. All the five senses are stimulated. The restless, wandering mind is calmed. Living, in all its protean forms, loses its "blur" and becomes more vivid and real. Experience suddenly assumes, as it were, a sharper focus.

In India and Tibet, there are almost as many different methods of breath control as there are gurus. Each teacher usually has developed his own modification of one of the many classical techniques described in the literature.

However, all methods, of whatever kind, are concerned with three phases of the breathing process: inhaling, holding the breath, and exhaling.

These three "moments" of the breath cycle must be harmonized by establishing the correct ratio among them.

Most people breathe irregularly. Their respiration is

affected by their state of health, work, smoking, alcohol, nervous tension, and so on.

Such an arrhythmia produces a wandering mind, moods of depression, lowered vitality; in fact, the kind of poor performance to be expected from any mechanism that needs a tune-up.

The pulse and rhythm of Nature

Wherever we look in nature, we find definite pulse and rhythm. The stars and planets in their courses, the seasons of the year, the migrations of birds and fish—each has its own predetermined cycle. Without such order and rhythm, creation would end in chaos.

Man, too, has his cycles, not only as time of life (infancy, youth, middle age, and autumn years), but also biological cycles. The latter involve physical stamina, power of concentration, intuition, and memory.

Some years ago, a German physician, Dr. William Fliess, began to wonder why a fever would suddenly come upon a patient and just as suddenly disappear. He initiated a close study of case histories in which this phenomenon was present. Gradually he came to the conclusion that these abrupt onsets and abatements followed a predictable cycle.

In fact, further research enabled him to determine the kind and duration of the basic biological cycles of man. He concluded that there are three distinct kinds of rhythm. One, he said, is a masculine cycle of 23 days' duration, which controls energy, aggressiveness, spirit of adventure, fighting instinct, physical strength and confidence.

Another periodicity, feminine in character, lasting 28 days, controls the intuition, feelings, moodiness, creative ability, artistic expression, and social sense.

A third cycle of 33 days, Dr. Fliess termed the intellectual rhythm, having faculties of both sexes: logic, memory, ambition, mental alertness, and concentration.

The German researcher gave the name biorhythm to these cycles, but students of Tantra will find in the general premise and description of the cycles a restatement of the *agamas*.

The qualities of the masculine cycle, for example, are precisely those of the *pingala* or sun breath. The feminine faculties are those of the *ida* or moon breath. And the intellectual cycle closely parallels the yogic *sushumna* flow, through the central spinal canal.

Indeed, in reporting the work of Dr. Fliess and his research associates, another writer declares:

"The gist of the problem lies in the bisexuality of man. The cell cycle—i.e., the discharge and regenerative period of the cell—is determined by the reciprocal action of male and female substances. Everyone is already familiar with one manifestation of this complex intrinsic process: the rhythmic ebb and flow of vitality." [2]

In learning breath control, the first requirement is to determine your individual rhythmic pulse as it is related to the pulsations of the earth.

The ratio of inhalation to exhalation and retention of breath varies from person to person and among different states of consciousness within the same person.

[2] Hans J. Wernli: "Biorhythm."

The average man normally takes fifteen breaths a minute, or 21,600 during each 24-hour period.

By speeding up or slowing down that respiratory rate, important changes, both physical and mental, occur.

Quick, shallow breathing is associated with excitement, anger, lust, alcohol, and so on. Yogis say that continuous rapid breathing produces a measure of anesthesia owing to the fact that the ego is forced partly out of the gross body into the subtle envelope (called *kosha*).

Prolonged rapid breathing (twenty to thirty breaths per minute) also produces heart palpitation and vertigo. More than one practicing physician has been awakened in the middle of the night by a patient who had suddenly awakened after a period of quick breathing in his sleep, and had imagined he was having a heart attack.

In such cases, it requires great persuasion and patience on the doctor's part to reassure the patient and to explain that the thudding of his heart was brought on by hyperventilation and not by a heart attack.

Thought control

Tantriks establish telepathic connection with any person whose thoughts they wish to control by noting the respiratory rate of that person. The number of breaths per minute is clearly evident in the rising and falling of the person's chest, as his diaphragm contracts and expands.

The yogi begins breathing at the same rate as that

of the person he wishes to reach. Within a short time, he establishes rapport with the other's inner consciousness and can mentally direct him.

Once "tuned in," the yogi can speed up or slow down the other person's breathing to produce whatever vibratory rate or state of consciousness may be desired.

"Brothers of the Shadows"

In passing, it should be pointed out that knowledge of this technique may be a dangerous blade that cuts two ways. The person whose breath cycle is being changed may be led into the deeper, slower rhythms of universal harmony and higher thoughts. On the other hand, he may be drawn downward into a state of restlessness, nervous euphoria, and sexual excitement.

Amongst those Tantriks who are called "brothers of the shadow," this insidious secret is sometimes used to achieve immoral ends.

Seven distinct breath cycles

Let us return, however, to the problem of determining one's own breath cycle.

Unfortunately, there is no precise rule of thumb for accomplishing this. The determination has to be made empirically.

After a little experimenting, the student should be able to find the rhythm and posture most natural and comfortable for him.

Secret Tantrik tradition teaches that there are seven distinct breaths, just as there are seven colors or rays of light in the spectrum, seven days of the week, seven planes of existence, and so on.

Accordingly, there are seven breathing techniques for the aspirant to practice in the preparatory stages of his *sadhana*.

Each exercise is practiced for a prescribed period of time before the aspirant proceeds to the next discipline. In India, where the pace of living is slower than it is in the West, the student practices at more frequent intervals and for a longer period of time than is practical for the occidental *Sadhaka*.

The more patience and dedication the student displays in laying the foundation of his yoga, the more satisfactory will be the results.

When practicing, it is not necessary for the Western student to torture his limbs into difficult *asanas* originally devised for people of a different culture—people who sit cross-legged most of their lives.

To be sure, some occidentals find that the postures described in books on Hatha Yoga come natural to them. For this fortunate, but small minority, the various yogic *asanas* may be assumed to good advantage, and without detracting from the more important phases of Tantrik *sadhana*.

For others, it is only necessary to assume a posture which is comfortable and which will hold the spine straight; and the chest, neck and head in a straight line.

This may be accomplished by sitting in a firm chair

in the attitude seen in sculptures of the ancient gods of Egypt.

In this stance, the heels should be placed about three inches apart, and the feet set at an angle to form a V.

When possible, the student faces a prescribed direction, depending usually upon the time of his practice. In the morning hours, he faces East; at noon, South; in the evening, West; and at midnight, due North.

FIRST DISCIPLINE

After assuming a comfortable posture, as described above, try to relax for a moment, and to empty the mind of cares and vexing trivia of the day.

Then exhale all the air in the lungs, drawing in the abdominal muscles to force out the residual air, which your customary shallow breathing allows to remain in the lungs.

Refill your lungs, drawing the air in very slowly, as you count up to seven. At that point, pause for a count of one, then again exhale slowly to the count of seven.

Repeat this cycle of 7:1:7 at least twelve times to clear the nasal passages and thus to make the next step in Tantrik methodology easier to perform.

Once the breath is flowing easily and rhythmically, inhale deeply (through both nostrils) and hold the breath in the mouth. Force it against the cheeks, making them bulge out. Hold the breath this way as long as possible without discomfort. Then expel the breath quickly and explosively through the mouth.

During the intake of air, mentally repeat the syllable

OM, and imagine that the breath flowing into your body carries with it a stream of cosmic life-force or *prana,* as indeed it does.

Further think of this vital current as circulating through the *nadis* or psychic channels of your subtle body and into the gross form, energizing every cell of your body.

The second breath, to be learned only after the first is fully mastered, is acquired as follows:

Go for a solitary walk, preferably in the open country or through a park, mountains, desert, woods, or along a seashore—where the air is fresh and unpolluted by industrial wastes.

As you stroll along, fully relaxed, inhale through both nostrils to the count of seven, as in the previous exercise. But this time, instead of holding the breath for one count, retain the breath for two counts. Then exhale to the count of seven once more—through the mouth. Hold the breath outside, that is, keep the lungs empty, for a count of two.

Repeat this breath cycle twelve times. After practicing it twice a day for three days, gradually increase the ratio from 7-2-7-2 to 10-5-10-5. That is, inhale through the nostrils to the count of ten; retain the breath for five counts; exhale to the count of ten; then hold the breath outside for five counts.

The third breath is sometimes called by Tantrik teachers the "measuring spoon" breath, owing to the manner in which the air is inhaled. The exercise is performed as follows:

With the lips parted slightly, as though about to pronounce the syllable "oo," inhale through the mouth in seven small draughts. Then swallow. Exhale through both nostrils to the count of seven. Repeat the cycle twenty-four times morning and evening for a week.

Man's fourth breath is known in India as the Lion Breath. It is executed thus:

Inhale through both nostrils to the count of four, or until the lungs are half filled. Then, retaining the breath, curl the tongue backward against the roof of the mouth, and emit a deep, growling sound: "Grrrrrr!"

The fifth breath should be effected in the open air, or near an open window. Purse the lips (and perhaps whistle the first few bars of a lively, familiar song). Then, keeping the lips in their puckered, whistling position, inhale slowly through the mouth to the count of seven. Pause for a single count, and exhale gently through both nostrils to the count of seven. Repeat the cycle six times. Practice this exercise morning and noonday.

The sixth breath is called the Serpent Breath, and is performed in this way:

With the tongue between the lips and protruding slightly, inhale through the mouth with a hissing sound. When the lungs are filled, hold the breath as long as it is comfortable to do so, then exhale slowly and uniformly through both nostrils. Repeat this pranayama five times in the morning and at noon and in the evening.

After practicing this exercise for two weeks, pass on to the seventh and final breath. First, exhale completely by drawing in the abdominal muscles to force the residual air from your lungs.

Close the right nostril with your right thumb, and slowly inhale through the left nostril. Do not overinflate your lungs. When filled to comfortable capacity, close also the left nostril.

(In India, the yogis have a prescribed method for closing the respective nostrils in pranayama. The index and middle fingers are folded downward into the palm, and the remaining two fingers are placed over the left nostril, while the thumb is used to close the right nostril. However, you may use whatever finger seems most natural to you.)

When you have filled your lungs and closed off both nostrils, hold the breath inside your lungs as long as possible without discomfort. When you first start to practice, the period of retention will not be long, but it will increase as you proceed, until you discover for yourself the *kumbhak* (interval of restraint) that belongs to your individual pranic rhythm.

When you begin to feel ill at ease, or a sense of suffocation, open the right nostril and, keeping the left closed, slowly exhale.

These three phases—inhalation (called *purak*), retention (*kumbhak*), and exhalation (*rechak*) constitute one complete cycle of breath control.

Repeat the cycle five times at each session during the first days of your practice. Then gradually increase the number to twelve.

This *pranayama* can be safely practiced several times a day if you are fortunate enough to have the time and privacy for it. Otherwise, once a day (morning or evening) will suffice.

You will feel, after each session, the results of your practice. The electro-magnetic pulses that flow through your entire body will calm and steady your mind, relax the muscles, and purify the blood stream.

These exercises constitute the first step in Tantrik methodology for the Western aspirant. Practice them for a minimum period of six weeks before going on to the more advanced exercises.

> "Forms, colors, densities, odors—what is it in me that
> corresponds with them?"
>
> WHITMAN: *"Leaves Of Grass"*

5. *Secret meaning of color*

Color, which has transformed man's environment and
has played a powerful but secret role in his inner life,
remains one of the least understood forces of today's
world.

For colors are but the various wave lengths of light.
And light is the mysterious alpha and omega of man's
existence.

In the remote past, primitive civilizations did not use
color as we do today, for its esthetic values. In ancient
Egypt, Chaldea, India and China, color was associated
with religious rites and with medicine.

"Evidence that the inspiring beauty of color had its origin in mysticism, in a sort of functional application of hue to interpret life and the world, and not in esthetics, piles high as we dig in the ruins of antiquity." [1]

Influence of color on sexual activity

In some of the early mystery schools of India and Persia, neophytes spent years exploring the profound nature and effects of a single color.

Now, after thousands of years, man is beginning to acquire a dim understanding of what color means to his life and personality.

The more original and independent researchers in medicine, physics, psychology, botany, and related sciences, have conducted experiments that have turned up "new" facts (known and used by Tantriks for centuries).

Scientists found, for example, that color significantly influences sexual activity. They discovered that violet light increases the activity of the female sex glands. Red light stimulates the male reproductive organs.

Likewise, it was learned that under red light, muscular tension increased from a normal of 23 units to 42 units. In orange light, tension further increased to 35 units. Yellow light produced 30 units, green 29, and blue 24.

Effect of color on the human mind was just as pronounced. Students bathed in a brilliant red light showed

1 Birren, Faber: "The Story of Color."

greater skill at solving mathematical problems than they did when exposed to ordinary light.

A "suicide bridge," long painted black, was changed to bright green. The death leaps immediately declined by one-third.

Further tests have shown that under an intense red light, a person will over-estimate the weight of objects. Conversely, under the influence of green light, objects appear to be lighter in weight than under ordinary illumination.

Distortion of the time sense has also been noted under colored light. Red and yellow make time seem to pass more slowly than ordinarily. Green and blue have the opposite effect: time appears to be accelerated.

In exploring the effects of color, scientists have noted that the degree to which any hue influences a person is partly determined by its quality, intensity and predominance; by the duration of one's exposure to it; by the age, sex, and race of the individual exposed.

Even in this space age, however, scientists as yet know nothing of the vast tides of cosmic color that daily flood the earth during their appointed periods, influencing all life upon this planet.

Only mystics and yogis know, and make use of, this knowledge.

In preparing for the secret ritual of *maithuna* or sex union, which forms the point of focus for Tantrik *sadhana,* and distinguishes it from other forms of yoga, the student uses color in the purification stage of his work.

Kaula adepts also use it in other and more powerful ways, of course. But its primary importance to the beginner is that of purifying the *nadis*, and of supplying them with new energy.

As previously noted, there are seven major centers of psychic force in man's subtle body—called *chakras*. Further, that each of these foci has a characteristic dominant color.

These major colors correspond to the seven visible rays of light that comprise the spectrum—namely, red, orange, yellow, green, blue, indigo and violet.

Since the *chakras* constitute part of the etheric body, the colors are not precisely those of the solar spectrum visible to us, but the resemblance is close enough for descriptive purposes.

In physics, it is well known that all these seven colors are merely different wave lengths of pure white light. Colored objects owe their individual hues to the fact that they absorb from the white light certain wave lengths, while they reflect or rediffuse others.

For example, in the case of an object such as a red ball, it is red because it absorbs all the light falling upon it except the red ray.

Similarly, in the subtle body, each *chakra* absorbs certain currents of vital solar energy, and rediffuses others.

Tantra teaches that the pure, all-pervading solar light is actually the primordial emanation of the divine being. It is the radiant energy released in the first "shining forth" of Shiva at the beginning of creation. All living creatures, from the highest *rishi* to the lowest microorganism, exist only so long as this Shiva energy (as *prana*) permeates their forms.

In man it is likewise this all-pervasive energy that vitalizes and links together the gross and subtle bodies, flowing freely from one to the other.

The physical manifestation of *prana* in animals is respiration. Breathing includes, again, both male and female principles. The inspiration or drawing in of the breath is of negative polarity and is feminine. Exhalation is positive and male.

As we shall see later, when we consider the meaning and effects of sound, the act of breathing in itself is considered by Hindus to be an inaudible prayer or *mantram*, even though it is uttered involuntarily. It is called the *ajapa mantram*.

The Shastra states that, as the divine current or solar breath is drawn into the body as we breathe, it makes the sound of "sah." When we exhale, that vibration forms the syllable, "hang."

Hence the frequent reference in Hindu texts to Hang-sah, meaning "the supreme *mantram*, the breath of God." It was, in fact, this breath that God breathed into Adam in the Biblical story of creation.

According to Tantra, the fiery star we know as the sun in reality veils from our physical sight the true spiritual sun, or God. And it is because they seek the divine Being behind the sun that many yogis in India stare fixedly at the dazzling orb until their eyes are burned out. Tantriks regard this form of search for reality a harmful and misguided *sadhana*.

It is this reverence for the spiritual sun as "the light and life of all things created," that inspired that most ancient and most important of all Hindu prayers, the Gayatri.

Today, as in centuries past, pious Hindus greet the dawn with the following mystical utterance:

"We meditate upon the unspeakable brilliance of

that resplendent Sun. May that direct our understanding."

To a person with only a superficial knowledge of Hinduism, such a prayer might appear a mere form of sun worship, a relic of some primitive religion of the past. How, they will ask, can solar radiation direct our understanding?

The answer, according to Shaktism, is that man receives from the sun certain kinds of energy that affect his mind as well as his body.

Science has identified in the sunlight of the earth's atmosphere minute particles that are charged with tremendous force. These are sometimes called vitality globules.

Almost everyone has had the experience of looking into the distance on a brilliant sunshiny day and of observing tiny, intensely bright specks of light, darting about in all directions. These are vitality globules. They are charged with a force that yogis call prana.

By absorbing these particles from the sunlight, we renew not only the vigor of our physical bodies, but of our subtle body as well.

It has been suggested [2] that depletion of vitality globules during a succession of cloudy days may account in part for lowered vitality during winter months of those who live in harsher climates.

Certainly, the aged and the convalescent know the importance of exposure to the warm, healing rays of bright sunshine.

The exact way in which simple light rays penetrate or affect the body is still a subject of research for science.

[2] Leadbeater, C. W.: "The Chakras."

One theory is that when color sensation is received through the eyes, the pituitary gland is stimulated, and secretes certain hormones. These pass directly into the blood stream and thus affect the body.

Some researches, on the other hand, have demonstrated beyond question that physical reaction to color can take place when the vision is completely sealed off.

One explanation advanced to account for this phenomenon states that the surface of the body possesses a radiation sense. The skin is believed to incorporate some kind of cells related to the nervous system. These cells perceive radiant energy, including the various frequencies of light.

Another opinion holds that the color rays, striking the surface of the body, set up corresponding vibrations within.

Those who are acquainted with the principles of Tantra say that the light enters the body through the six chakras or plexuses of the etheric double, described elsewhere.

Particularly concerned with this process is the *svadisthana* chakra, situated in the area of the generative organs. The vitality globule is drawn into the epicenter of this chakra, where its seven atoms are separated and diffused into seven currents, each of a different color.

Six of these color rays radiate outward along the six *nadis* or spokes of the plexus, while the seventh is absorbed into the center itself.

Thus the rose-red indraught of the sun is diffused throughout the body, stimulating the nervous system and vitalizing the entire organism.

The orange ray seeks out the root chakra at the base

of the spine. There it stimulates the sex glands and energizes the etheric body.

The yellow ray pours into the abdominal region of the body, and is polarized in the *manipura* chakra. It stimulates the adrenals, pancreas, and liver.

The green ray is directed to the *anahata* center, affecting the region of the heart, or cardiac plexus. It gives balance and harmony to the body.

The current of blue energy surges upward to the throat. It is cooling, ethereal and spiritual. It influences the thyroid gland.

The indigo beam floods the area of the brow chakra between the eyebrows. It affects the pineal gland and is related to paranormal faculties such as telepathy and clairvoyance.

Finally, the violet ray from the vitality globule refraction is directed to the coronal force center or *sahasrara,* just above the crown of the head. Its influence in the gross body is expressed through the pituitary gland.

It is important to remember at this point that all the vital energy discussed in the preceding paragraphs has but a single source—the sun.

To the Tantrik this means that all the various frequencies of light we have been discussing are of the Shiva principle. And since the aim of all Shakta practice is the marriage of the two polar streams—Shiva and Shakti—the Tantrik seeks to unite the energy of the sun with that from another source.

Kundalini, the Shakti power, is not derived directly from the atmosphere, as is the solar energy. Rather, it comes from "the womb of Shakti," deep within the earth; from the very core of our planet, where rages an inferno whose temperatures rival those of the sun itself.

But the Agamas point out that this primary force from below is a wholly different kind of energy from that radiated by the sun.

The solar prana is dynamic power, which diffuses itself throughout the body, vitalizing every cell, down to the most microscopic.

Kundalini or "serpent fire," on the other hand, is normally static—sealed off, so to speak, at the base of the spine. Once released and set in motion, it must be controlled or it can ravage body, mind and spirit.

The aim of the Tantrik is to direct the centripetal Shakti force upward to the higher centers, there to complete union with the centrifugal Shiva energy.

Warnings

But the literature is full of warnings to the uninitiated that, if not properly controlled, the aroused kundalini may rush downward, bringing union with a lower order of creation.

The carnal appetites are then vastly intensified. Worldly ambitions are likewise stimulated, together with the will to satisfy them at any cost. Lust, anger, greed—the whole catalog of evil passions—take over.

When the fiery Shakti current rises, however, and is led upward by the yogi, it gathers momentum as it ascends the central canal of the spine, piercing chakra after chakra, until the highest is attained.

A polarization of the two—Shiva and Shakti—then takes place.

"On their union, nectar (*amrita*) flows which, in an ambrosial stream, runs from the *Brahma-rudhra* to the *muladhara*, flooding the microcosm. It is then that the sadhaka, forgetful of all in this world, is immersed in ineffable bliss. Refreshment, increased power and enjoyment, follow upon each visit to the well of life." [3]

However, our immediate concern is with prana, the seven-rayed emanation from the sun. Greater absorption of vitality globule energy through the chakras is one of the objectives of Tantrik discipline. It is accomplished through chromatic pranayama or color breathing.

The procedure is quite simple. Its effectiveness depends to some extent upon the intensity with which the student can visualize the various colors, drawing them in from the universal radiation and causing them to flood the various areas of the body.

SECOND DISCIPLINE

If possible, practice this exercise between the hours of 9:30 a.m. and noon.

It should be performed before an open window and preferably in full sunlight.

Seated in a comfortable posture, as described in the first discipline, face the East. Close your eyes, and for a few moments try to feel the luminous radiant energy pouring over you in a life-giving flood. Realize that the seven rays of color that fill space also penetrate the psychic centers of your etheric body, and permeate every cell and tissue of your physical body.

[3] Avalon, Arthur: "The Serpent Power."

Then relax, allowing your whole frame to go limp.

After a moment, sit upright and exhale all the air from the lungs, forcing it out by drawing in the abdomen.

Inhale slowly to the count of seven, expanding the abdomen. Hold the breath, as you count from one to seven, at the same time strongly willing and visualizing the color red. Imagine that it flows over the lower portion of the stomach and the genitals; then mentally picture it covering the back of your head.

Exhale to the count of seven. Pause one second. Then repeat the breath cycle, visualizing red as before. Perform the red pranayama three times.

Then, as you inhale for the fourth cycle, imagine the color yellow deluging the area of the upper chest and forehead. Carry the yellow awareness through three breath cycles, as in the case of red.

Do the same with blue, envisioning that color as a cool, healing spiritual effulgence in the area of the throat, solar plexus, and top of the head. It will bring serenity and poise.

Finally, after the one-second pause between breaths, repeat the pranayama, mentally infusing the feet, legs, arms, and face with a pure white radiance.

This discipline ought to be practiced twelve times before proceeding to the next.

The Shastra repeatedly reminds the student that patient attention to details of these early and basic disciplines will be the measure of your success in later undertakings.

"The merging of mind is achieved by listening to inner sound."

—*Hatha Yoga Pradipika*

6. *Hidden power of sound*

We dwell not only in an ocean of light (color), but of sound as well.

Vast tides of this vibrational energy, which Tantriks call *nadam,* flow around and through all things—living and non-living, visible and invisible.

The Shastra teaches that even before there was light at the dawn of creation, God's first manifestation was *shabda,* a sound or word.

Christian scripture expresses the same view. John, the beloved disciple, wrote:

"In the beginning was the Word, and the Word was with God, and the Word was God." [1]

The Divine Mother who sings the Symphony of the Universe

Thus, as the creative fiat of God, *shabda* or sound vibration is present everywhere. It expresses itself in a million different ways, from the "music of the spheres," to all the cacophony of man's society. Tantriks say that it is the Divine Mother who sings the symphony of the universe, "the beginning of which is creation, and the conclusion is dissolution."

In the industrialized West, the omnipresent sounds that assault our ears seem less the voice of God than the infernal din of the devil.

Most of us spend our lives amidst a vast pandemonium of harsh sounds, which science has shown are greatly detrimental to both health and peace of mind.

Experiments made in the course of various noise abatement campaigns in all our large cities have revealed that the constant repetition of strident and penetrating noises actually produces lasting damage to the nervous system and to the various organs of the body affected by it.

Stomach ulcers, hypertension, degenerative diseases of the arteries and nervous exhaustion are just a few of the common ailments that science now attributes in part to our noisy environment.

1 John I:1.

Those of us who dwell in large cities are exposed around the clock to traffic uproar, sirens, pneumatic drills, blaring speakers of neighborhood radio and TV sets, airplanes overhead, and so on.

Researchers tell us that the respective vibrations from these sources reach us in the form of waves transmitted through the air, and that our brains are constantly at work sorting and identifying them, even though we are not consciously aware of it.

They state that urban residents today have not the faintest idea of what the word quiet means.

For example, ordinary street sounds and background noise during an average day in any city will usually measure 40 or 50 decibels.

Compare this with the same day in the country, where the gentle rustling of leaves measures only 10 decibels.

The true implications of a noisy environment may be forcibly brought home to the reader when he considers the fact that the automobile horn, to which he is exposed during most of his waking hours, produces an average noise level of 90 decibels (10 to 15 feet away from the source).

Tests have clearly established that a noise of 90 decibels causes the amount of blood pumped through the heart to double.

Yet recent surveys have revealed that in large cities, traffic noises are increasing from year to year. After conducting on-site studies, one sound engineer declared that:

"A person standing on the corner of 42nd Street and Fifth Avenue in New York City, where, in business hours the noise level fluctuates between 60 and 75 decibels, is for the moment just as badly off in audition as a person of defective hearing whose threshold in the middle range of frequencies is 45 to 60 decibels above normal. He has lost 25 to 35 percent of normal hearing." [1]

It is evident, however, that this state of existence is wholly acceptable to the city dweller, who is unaware of the ravages being wrought on his person. So accustomed is he, in fact, to the deafening background of his life that the quiet, low-decibel sounds of the country are painful and terrifying to him.

One New Yorker who went to the country for "a little rest and quiet," soon hastened back to the roaring metropolis. He complained bitterly of being awakened early in the morning by "those damned birds screaming on the window-sill."

In our day, the terrifying destructive power of sound extends much further than mere background noise in our cities, however.

Residents of areas near military airfields have had some intimation of the formidable power of sound. Jet bombers, in supersonic power dives at low altitudes, produce shock waves that resemble bomb blasts. Moreover, they produce visible damage in the form of shattered windows and broken dishes.

Dr. Heinz Gartman, a German scientist whose field is jet propulsion and aero engines, observed:

"We may imagine the consequences if a Hustler (a large jet bomber) were permitted to roar across the country at supersonic speeds while remaining at low altitudes. A path of destruction 1000 feet wide would mark its route. Gusts of hurricane force would smash

[1] Mills, John: "A Fugue In Cycles and Bels."

houses, vehicles, ships; would mow frightful swaths through fields, orchards and woods; would wreak destruction wherever it passed. Imagine utilizing such a weapon over a crowded highway." [2]

A California scientist, Dr. Leo Baranski, was recently quoted as saying that the idea of destroying an object by intensifying its frequency could lead to satellite-borne weapons, tuned to frequencies of concrete and steel, which would disintegrate cities.

On the biopositive or constructive side, Dr. Baranski believes that experiments now under way may lead to doubling man's lifespan. This would be accomplished, he said, by using resonant frequency to stimulate a finger-sized area at the top of the spinal cord.

Situated at this point is an organ known as the medullary mitochondria, which produces a substance called adenosine-triphosphatase (ATP for short), that is released throughout the body. Molecules of this substance have a peculiar ability to absorb photons (the vitality globules previously discussed) from the sun, and to store them in food.

By using the proper sound frequency, concentrated at this point, Dr. Baranski believes the ATP molecules should release greater amounts of free energy than they now do.

"Controlled release of ATP's energy, with brief bursts of radiation, could mean incredible strength of mind and body to meet emergencies," he said.

Tantrik literature contains many passages which, in different terminology, state theories quite similar to that of Dr. Baranski.

[2] Gartmann, Heinz: "Man Unlimited."

One text declares: "The manifest sound of God (Shabdabrahman) exists in all things as consciousness. So it is this sound, the substance of which is consciousness, which exists in the bodies of living beings in the form of kundalini; and then appears as letters in prose, poetry and so forth, being carried by the psychic current to the throat, teeth, and other places." [3]

Hindu teachers of antiquity held that the gibberish of a child just learning to talk is not due to his imperfect imitation of words he hears, but to an obstruction of the main *nadi* or subtle channel leading from the root chakra to the throat.

When, through obstruction of the vocal passage, a child utters indistinct sounds, it is the kula-kundalini who, playing in the aperture of the *muladhara* and coiled around sushumna, utters indistinct sounds repeatedly. It is the echo of this indistinct sound which issues from the passage of a child's throat.[4]

Elsewhere it is written that the same obstruction or "defilement" occurs also at death. "At the beginning of Japa (breathing), a devotee is affected by birth uncleanliness, and at the end of Japa by death uncleanliness." [5]

Words—or more precisely, the individual letters that comprise them—are nothing more than the mysterious kundalini, given articulate form in speech or symbolized in writing.

As the supreme energy of Brahman, brought to manifestation in speech, language has for the Tantrik both a wonderful and a terrifying significance.

Each letter of the alphabet is a *mantram*, that is, a sound vibration of given frequency, which produces its

[3] The Sharadatilaka.   [4] Prapanyaca-sara.
[5] Kularnava Tantra.

own shape in the ether. In ancient India, there were rishis or great seers who claimed they could see the shapes thus produced in the *akasha* (ether of space). They taught that, since these sound forms or etheric doubles of universal objects were imperishable, words are also imperishable.

In a modern study of how sounds can produce definite forms or structures, experimenters have made use of a technical invention called an eidophone. A plastic, paste-like mixture was spread over the surface of a diaphragm. When words were spoken underneath it, it was found that vocal sound waves created beautiful floral shapes—trees, flowers, and leaf fronds.

Similar experiments have been conducted with musical sounds, both as to their form and their colors.

Sages of antiquity developed an extensive vocabulary of secret words of power, formed from Sanskrit syllables. The most widely known, most powerful and basic of these is, of course, the mystic syllable OM.

Patanjali, the great Indian pundit who codified the systems of yoga two centuries before Christ, stated that the repetition of OM invokes Isvara, the supreme God.

According to Tantrik texts, the sound-form of OM embraces all creation. It is everywhere, in all things, manifest or unmanifest. Properly intoned, it will produce harmony and balance in body and mind.

In passing, it is interesting to note that Indian tradition regards only the original Vedic idiom as valid for mantra making. The sacred literature asserts that the entire cosmos was evolved out of fifty *bija mantras* or seed sounds. These sounds were revealed to the early rishis during deep spiritual states and came from God's own mind.

From their subtle matrices the process of evolution brought forth etheric centers of force around which revolve molecules and atoms that form visible and dense matter.

So it is said: "The particular letters and number of letters which God has ordained should convey a particular meaning, and are capable of conveying that meaning do, when uttered successively in the manner prescribed, convey that meaning." [6]

Later non-Vedic languages are regarded as merely conversions or permutations of the substantive Sanskrit.

Few modern authorities on linguistics agree with this view, although some notable scholars have indicated that there may be some truth in it.

Sir William Jones, one of the first Westerners to make a thorough and critical study of Sanskrit, wrote:

"The Sanskrit language, whatever be its antiquity, is of a wonderful structure; more perfect than the Greek, more copious than the Latin, and more exquisitely refined than either; yet bearing to both of them a stronger affinity, both in the roots of verbs and in the forms of grammar, than could possibly have been produced by accident; so strong, indeed, that no philologer could examine them all three without believing them to have sprung from some common source, which perhaps no longer exists." [7]

Be that as it may, Tantrik ritual holds strictly to the seminal Matrika-shakti or fifty Sanskrit letters, from A to Ksa, as being the primary manifestation of kundalini, "the seed of all things moving or non-moving.[8]

6 Tantra Tattva.
7 Sir William Jones: "Works, Vol. ii."
8 Kamadhenu Tantra.

The letters are called *varnas,* which means colors, because each has its own vibrational hue. Some are red, some of a brilliant electric blue, some white, and so on.

They are, of course, as the gurus of antiquity have said, to be considered merely the outward or gross expression of the more subtle aspect of sound, which is consciousness itself. For this reason, Tantrik writings refer to lettered and unlettered sound.

The unlettered or subtle aspect of sound is said to flow inside the body as currents of vital energy, owing to the movement of prana, as we inhale and exhale in breathing. That is why, as previously stated, breathing itself is called *ajapa mantram* or unrecited prayer.

Even though sound is outwardly expressed from the vocal organs, it is not generated there, according to Shaktism. Instead, it appears first at the opening of the *muladhara* or root chakra, where it makes a faint, murmuring sound, like the humming of a swarm of bees. In the Satchakra Tattva, it is written: "She it is whose sweet constant murmuring and humming, sounds like that of a swarm of black bees, intoxicated with a draught of honey."

This extremely subtle state of sound, called *para* in Hindu texts, goes unperceived by the ordinary person. Its energy moves upward within the central *nadi* of the spine to the *anahata* chakra in the region of the heart. There, says the Vishvasara Tantra, is produced the "unstruck sound."

"It is here that the Syllable of Obeisance—OM—is manifested, here that the living self stands like a lamp in a windless spot."

Om, the sacred syllable which exists in this silent place of the heart, is the greatest of all words of power.

Ancient seers declared it to be representative of the highest aspect of God. When properly recited by the aspirant, its secret meaning is gradually understood and liberation results.

Continuing upward through the central channel, the vibrational energy of Shiva is transferred into a gross state. It is as the latter that it issues from the throat in the form of articulate sound.

Such sound may assume any modulation: speech, wordless cry, grunt, groan, etc. Regardless of the way in which it is expressed, it is the supreme consciousness of God, issuing as gross sound.

Some schools of Shaktism assert that the quality of this sound in man—that is, speech—is an indication of his stage of spiritual development or condition of life.

One of the first signs that yogic practice has borne fruit is said to be a pleasant and resonant voice. The theory is that as the sadhaka purifies himself through practice, the sound energy within him comes to resemble more closely the creative harmony of Mantra-shakti or divine sound.

Learning to hear the inner, "unstruck sound" is in itself a creative act. It forms one of the most important of the Tantrik disciplines. For, "leaving all thoughts and all strivings, meditating upon sound alone, his mind merges into sound," [9] finally to pass beyond into the ether of pure consciousness.

Tantrik gurus differ according to their respective schools as to the number of ways the aspirant must perceive inner sound. Some say seven, others ten.

These sounds have been likened unto those of the

[9] Nadabindu Upanishad.

ocean, thunder, waterfall, clinking of tiny silver chains, a swarm of bees, rustling of leaves, a huge drum, shrill whistling, a bell, a flute, a conch, humming of a wire or a stringed instrument.

There is no prescribed order in which these various states of inner sound may appear to the yogi. Authorities say it depends upon the advancement of the individual, that is, whether he has practiced yoga in former lives, and so on.

However, most adepts agree that the first sounds perceived are more plenary and intense, such as the ocean's roar, thunder, or a bass drum. As the sadhaka advances with practice, the sounds become musical: bells, a stringed instrument, a flute. Finally, as inner attunement becomes more refined, the yogi perceives directly the subtle modes of cosmic sound, like distant tinkling of bells, a lute, a bee.

"Thus are the many sounds heard, growing more and more refined. Even when the louder sounds like that of a big drum are heard, the yogi should continue to listen to the subtler ones."

In India and Tibet, several methods of listening to inner sound are taught, but the following are probably the most suitable for Western students:

THIRD DISCIPLINE

The Shastra prescribes the post-midnight hours for the practice of this discipline.

The sadhaka first retires to a place of comparative quiet, where outside sounds will not distract him as he begins to concentrate upon the inner sound.

Seated in a comfortable position, facing either East or North, he calms his mind by *japa mantra,* that is, by breathing in and out rhythmically, while mentally repeating the sacred syllable Om. Inhalation should be to the count of seven. Hold one count. Exhale seven. Hold one; inhale, etc.

The mystic syllable is repeated mentally one hundred and eight times in this way. For keeping count of the breaths, the Yogini Tantra recommends a rosary of one hundred and eight beads. These may be of *rudrakshas* (seeds of a plant employed in Shiva rites) or of pearls, crystals, gold, silver, coral; or of shells.

After the thoughts are stilled, the sadhaka gazes steadily, without blinking, at some fixed point (such as a candle flame) on a level with the eyes, and four or five feet away. As he looks, without winking, at this point, he listens intently for the inner sound in his right ear.

To achieve more intense concentration, after gazing at the point for a minute or more, he may close his eyes.

Even though the first three or four sessions may not yield satisfactory results, the sadhaka is instructed to persist in his practice for at least a week.

At the end of that period, if he feels the need for more concrete results, he may try the method known as *yoni mudra,* which is performed as follows:

Seated in an erect posture, rest the elbows on a pillow or cushion placed before you on a table or desk top. Place the thumbs lightly upon the tragus (small flaps) of the ears, thus closing them to exterior sounds. Close your eyes with the index fingers. Press the lips together between the remaining two fingers. Then breathe slowly and gently through the nose. Meanwhile, concentrate the attention solely upon sounds to be heard in the closed ears.

After some practice, the student will find that his mind is more and more absorbed in the sounds, so that he forgets his body, senses and thoughts. He loses himself in the vast sea of sound vibrating throughout the universe. The two polar streams of creation—male and female, Shiva and Shakti—will unite in the ultimate harmony of being.

It is the echo of man's yearning, which sounds even unto the realm of eternal life.

> "The Seal of Musk: for this let those pant who pant for bliss."
>
> —*The Koran*

7. *Fragrance of being*

From the dust of the earth to the spirit of man that inhabits it, there is nothing completely odorless in creation.

Each of us exudes his own individual scent, which dogs, mystics and ordinary persons endowed with a keen sense of smell can recognize instantly.

The kind and intensity of the odor that surrounds us depend upon a number of factors: state of health, cosmetics, spiritual advancement, even our thought patterns.

Literature, both East and West, contains many references to the "odor of sanctity." An oft-quoted saying in India is that "The fragrance of a flower travels with the wind, but the odor of sanctity travels against the wind."

Similarly, early Christian historians have recorded the specific smells associated with various saints. Thus, it is said that St. Francis of Assisi smelled of lemon; St. Cajetan of orange blossoms; St. Catherine of violets; St. Trevere of lilies; St. Rose of the flower of the same name; St. Teresa of jasmine and orris root; and St. Lydwine of cinnamon.

An evil life exhales its own peculiar nidor, too, just as the saintly one does perfume. The famous French detective, Vidocq once declared:

"Put me in a crowd of a thousand persons, and by the sense of smell alone, I will single out every violator of the moral law."

He maintained that every branch of the criminal profession has its own odor, and that he had learned to identify each one.

For the most part, however, the mysteries of scent, which were explored so fully by the ancients, have been left largely to commercial chemists and to cosmeticians in Western lands.

Scientific research as well as the fine arts have provided us with a considerable body of knowledge concerning our auditory, tactile, visual and gustatory faculties. Only the sense of smell remains unexamined.

This is somewhat surprising when we consider the important role the perfumer's art has played in the history of mankind.

The oldest means of influencing man's two deepest instincts

Odor is perhaps the oldest means of influencing man's two deepest instincts: sex and religion. And by means of these primary drives, in turn, it has determined the destiny of empires and governments, the individual fate of king and commoner alike.

Knowing the secret power of perfumes, the priests and sorcerers of ancient civilizations compounded unguents and precious ointments so powerful that the fragrance of some of them has endured for thousands of years. Sealed jars and vases of alabaster and onyx, found in the tombs of Egyptian Pharaohs and recently opened, have yielded the balmy aroma of spikenard and balsam.

Scholars are agreed that the earliest use of pleasing odors was probably religious. Incense and burnt offerings as a part of religious rites dates back to remote times. Egyptians, Chaldeans, Hebrews, Greeks, Romans —all believed that the smoke of sweet-smelling gums and spices, ascending heavenward from their altars, would delight the gods.

Hence the very name perfume, derived from the Latin "per fumum," meaning by or through fumes.

Close relationship of sexual and religious passions

Priests of those ancient cultures were aware that the aromatic substances used in religious ceremonies not only pleased the gods, but also influenced the worshippers' state of mind.

Noting this fact, a modern writer recently observed:

"This mental disposition (religious fervor) is to a great extent due to the inhalation of the volatilized terebinthinate constituents of the incense, which produces an obscure yet perceptibly stimulant effect on the erection center; *were the effect stronger, it would excite distinct erotic emotions with erection,* but as it is, it only produces religiously devotional emotions, arguing, however, the close relationship of our sexual and our religious passions." [1] (Italics mine)

In Hebrew scripture, it is God Himself who commands Moses to "make an altar to burn incense upon." After setting forth the exact dimensions and materials to be used in construction of the altar, Jehovah instructs him to have Aaron burn incense upon it each evening when he lights the lamps. "He shall burn incense upon it, a perpetual incense before the Lord throughout your generations." [2]

God also gave to Moses the formula for a holy anointing oil to be used in consecrating Aaron and his sons to the priesthood.

This use of perfumed anointing oil was later extended to rites investing monarchs with "the divine right of kings" at coronation ceremonies.

In June 1953, more than 3500 years after the time of Moses, Elizabeth II was anointed with holy oil, marking her ascension to the throne of England.

The formula of the oil so used is a closely guarded secret. However, at the time of the Queen's coronation,

1 Wall, O. A., M.D.: "Sex and Sex Worship."
2 Exodus 30:8.

an article published in the British trade magazine, "Pharmaceutical Journal," listed some of the oil's components. They were: essential oils of orange flowers, roses, cinnamon, jasmine and sesame; together with benzoin, musk, civet, and ambergris.

According to the Journal's editor, "the oil has a rich and peculiar fragrance: it is amber-coloured when freshly made, but time deepens the colour, and the odour becomes mellow and rare."

Outside the temple and palace, perfumes for centuries have been used in all countries for secular purposes as well.

The most common use, of course, has been that of scenting the body and clothing. This is done ostensibly for esthetic reasons. In actuality, however, the underlying motive has always been that of sex stimulation and sex allure.

This fact is nowhere more evident than in historical accounts of great courtesans and enchantresses. Jezebel, Messalina, Delilah, Thais, Phryne, Cleopatra, Empress Josephine—literature both sacred and profane is replete with stories of women whose strange power over men owed much to the magic art of perfumery.

Plutarch tells how Cleopatra used perfume to ensnare Antony and "to awaken and kindle to fury passions that as yet lay still and dormant in his nature."

He goes on to describe how her famous barge with gilded stern, outspread purple sails and silver oars came sailing up the river Cyndas to meet Antony for the first time. People along the shore were enveloped with clouds of perfume that were wafted from her vessel as it glided by.

In his play, "Antony and Cleopatra," Shakespeare says of the Nile Queen:

"She was so perfumed that the winds were lovesick."

Perfume ingredients as related to the sexual functions of animals or plants

That the olfactory sense can be used to arouse deep-rooted natural desires is not surprising when one considers that the essential ingredients of most perfumes are related to the sexual function of animals or plants.

For example, musk, the animal perfume whose popularity dates from the very dawn of civilization, is obtained from a gland developed by the male deer as a sex lure.

Darwin states that the gland and its secretion represent a powerful end-product of natural selection. Beginning ages ago, the male deer who exuded the muskiest scent attracted more females than those less abundantly endowed. As a consequence, he left a greater number of descendants. These, in turn, were subject to the same principle of natural selection, with descendants producing glands that were more and more potent.

Today, a single grain of musk can perfume several million cubic feet of air without any noticeable reduction in its size.

As the knowledge of musk and its aphrodisiac properties spread, the demand for it grew—especially among kings, rajahs, sybarites and courtesans.

It was the favorite scent of Empress Josephine, who

always carried a lace handkerchief impregnated with it. It is said that she used so much of it to inflame Napoleon's passion that the walls of her apartment exuded the fragrance for years afterward.

Historians similarly report that Henry IV of France could date his infatuation with Gabrielle d'Estrees from the moment she handed him her musk-saturated handkerchief to wipe his brow during a dance in a warm ballroom.

Biologists and students of human behavior have put forward the theory that in remote times, scent was the primary attraction between the sexes. They believe that other, and more refined, relationships evolved later. With the development of these more sophisticated attractions, scent receded into the background.

But they tell us that buried deep within the human organism is an atavistic response to the same animal odor that attracts the female deer.

Even floral perfumes are related to what Tantriks call the Shiva-Shakti play of nature. The oil glands of the flowers are for the purpose of effecting fecundation. A large portion of the essential oil is consumed during the process of fertilization. Once generation has been accomplished, the remaining fragrant essences recede into the stem and are diffused through other organs of the plant.

Horticulturists who grow flowers for use by perfumers know this, and are careful to harvest their crops just before fertilization occurs. In that way, they reap the blossoms at the time they are most fully laden with essential oils.

Various scents evoke responses other than sexual, of course. These, however, are largely due to past associations and are somewhat subjective. The emotion stimulated by an odor for one person is not always the same as that for another.

Some generalizations have nevertheless been attempted. Thus, it is said that the scent of magnolia may stimulate the fighting instinct. That of cloves is believed to be conducive to suspicion and gossip. Bergamont is reported to put one in a thoughtful or meditative frame of mind, ambergris fosters the art of poetry. And, for some obscure reason, ancient writers believed the lemon-like scent of verbena incited men to drunkenness.

In India, incense and fragrant essences still figure in all Hindu rites of worship. The odor of *dhoop* and *dhoona* floats from every shrine and temple in daily use.

But most Tantriks use certain scents in a more personal and more conducive way. Their primary aim is to stimulate the muladhara or root chakra, where kundalini energy lies coiled. For this subtle center is directly related to the sense of smell, and is easily influenced by certain aromas.

Accordingly, Tantriks (especially the *vamacharis*) employ specified essential oils in the manner prescribed for them by their individual gurus.

In general, the scents used in these rites are one or more of the following: musk, jasmine (champak), patchouli, spikenard, sandalwood and saffron.

Members of some of the more obscure sects of Kaulas anoint different parts of the body of their *mudra* (ritual sex partner) with different perfumes. Oil of jasmine is used for the hands, patchouli for the cheeks and breasts, spikenard for the hair, musk for the *mons veneris*, sandalwood for the thighs, and saffron for the feet.

For most Shaktas, however, a far simpler procedure is

followed, as we shall see in the chapter detailing the secret ritual, that is, the ultimate rite of Tantrism, which culminates in *maithuna* or ceremonial sex union.

Musk and patchouli (or perfumes having them as the dominant note) are the scents most commonly used in the Panchatattva or rite of the "five true things."

Synthetic perfumes are never used for these rites. In India and Tibet, of course, the simple essence or extract is always available from the local *gundhi* or perfume seller in any bazaar. In the case of musk, it is—as it should always be—greatly diluted. Allusion has already been made to the minute amount of musk needed to perfume a whole room. Moreover, in its pure form, it is tremendously expensive, selling for about $40,000 a pound.

Several years ago, Dr. Wallace Carrothers, a Du Pont research chemist, synthesized musk as astrotone. This and other synthetics, as previously pointed out, are not acceptable for Tantrik rites.

In Western countries, musk extract and oil of *patchouli* are obtainable from firms which supply perfume manufacturers.

Again, it should be borne in mind that the chief reason for using scent in Tantrik *sadhana* is the stimulation of the root chakra. The fact that scents so used are aphrodisiac merely points up that sexual libido and the energy of Shakti are one and the same.

> "O mistress of Kula! in Kuladharma enjoyment becomes complete yoga; bad deeds are made good deeds, and the world becomes the seat of Liberation."
>
> —*Kularnava Tantra*

8. *The five true things*

Opponents of Tantra—and they are many—almost always base their denunciation solely upon the fact that the system includes ritual drinking and sexual rites.

Censure of this kind is not new, if we are to believe accounts given in ancient literature itself.

For example, according to the Chinachara-sara Tantra, the great Indian sage, Vashistha, son of Brahma, was told to seek out Vishnu in the body of Buddha, and to be initiated by him.

Vashishtha accordingly entered Mahachina (probably Tibet), a land which the text says was inhabited by thousands of beautiful young girls "whose hearts were gladdened with wine." It adds that "the movement of their hips made their girdles of little bells tinkle."

Vashishtha is surprised and outraged to find Buddha, "his eyes drooping from wine," in the midst of this erotic revelry.

"These are practices contrary to the Vedas!" he cries. "I do not approve of it!"

But a voice out of space tells him:

"If you wish to gain my grace speedily, this is the way it must be done."

A similar story is told concerning the celebrated guru, Padma Sambhava, who introduced Buddhism into Tibet.

One of Padma's friends visited him at his cemetery retreat, where he found him living with a female disciple named Mandarava.

"What a fine example you are!" he told Padma. "You left your lawful wife Bhasadhara in your palace in the Urgyan country; and this is quite disgraceful!"

The account goes on to say that Padma thought to himself: "Inasmuch as this fellow is ignorant of the inner significance of the Mahayana and of the yogic practices pertaining to the three chief psychic channels, I should pardon him."

In modern times, even as enlightened a preceptor as Madame Blavatsky failed to grasp the true meaning and methods of Tantrism. As a consequence, she defined Durga or Kali (the dynamic form of Shakti energy) as "the special energy connected with sexual rites and magical powers—the worst form of black magic or sorcery." [1]

1 Blavatsky, Helena: "Theosophical Glossary."

Her latter-day disciple, Guy de Purucker, followed her example. In his "Occult Glossary," he characterizes the Tantras as "heirlooms handed down from originally debased or degenerate Atlantean racial offshoots."

"There is," he admits, "a certain amount of profoundly philosophical and mystical thought running through the more important Tantrik works, but the Tantrik worship in many cases is highly licentious and immoral."

It is true that some of the more extreme Kaula rites—especially as practiced in Assam and parts of Tibet—would be shocking to the Western student.

Also, the liturgy of many of the Tibetan Tantrik schools has a weird and somewhat frightening sound to occidental ears. This is more particularly true of ceremonies involving deities in their destructive or terrifying aspects.

Invocation to Zhing-Skyong

The following invocation to Zhing-Skyong, Tibetan guardian of cemeteries, is typical. It is contained in a Tibetan blockprint written by the monk Tikshanti and published at the Krashi Lungpo Lamasary:

"To the south of Bodhgaya (in India) is situated the great cemetery, Silba'i Tshal. At this supreme place, one can hear the mighty voices of the gShin Rje (demons), the magically powerful howling of the *ma mo,* the splashing of the sea of blood, the sputtering of the lamps fed with human fat. There is visible also the coiling smoke, rising from the evil burnt offering. There sounds the thudding of the male *bdud* (ferocious figures) who are dancing a drum dance; and the whirling of the femal *bdud*, who turn in a ring dance; the blaring of the thigh-bone trumpets, the roar of wild animals. There is visible the quick flaring up of the great scorching lightnings; there is audible the fierce rolling thunder and the crashing of great yellow meteors. The horrible laughter of the multitude of *bdud* and *yakshas* causes the earth foundations to quake." [2]

To the reader uninitiated in *sandha-bhasa* or the secret language of Tantrism, such a description must seem like a brief but terrying glimpse into hell.

In any case, to evaluate all Tantrik thought and practice in terms of its extreme sects, is like judging all Christianity by the dukhobors or the flagellants.

Physical, social, mental and moral fitness to practice the secret ritual

Critics who condemn Tantrism because of its use of the sex force as an underlying constant are ignorant of, or choose to ignore a basic tenet of Shaktism—one which precedes and governs the so-called fifth tattva or mystical coition.

That prerequisite is called *adhikara,* meaning competency or fitness to practice the secret ritual. The Shastra is explicit in stating that each aspirant should

2 Nebesky-Wojkowitz translation.

undertake only that stage of initiation for which he is prepared. It expressly forbids the pashu or person of predominantly carnal appetites to indulge in *lata-sadhana*, the discipline requiring sexual intercourse.

Almost without exception, Tantrik scriptures, both Indian and Tibetan, specify in detail the postulant's qualifications: physical, social, mental and moral.

Thus the Gautamiya Tantra declares that the disciple should be "of good parentage, pure-minded and possessing a strong physique and sound mind. He should be one who has conquered passions, indolence, illusory knowledge and anger."

The Gandharva Tantra likewise states that the person seeking this kind of initiation "must be intelligent, senses controlled, abstaining from injury to all beings, ever doing good to all, pure, a believer. . . ."

Specifically rejected (for example, in the Kularnava Tantra, Ch. 13) are "the glutton, lecher, shameless, greedy, ignorant, hypocrite, voluptuary and drunkard."

Both the Matsya-Shukta Tantra and the Maharu-draya-mala make similar proscriptions, adding the slothful and the irreligious.

It is noteworthy, in fact, that all Tantrik schools make belief in God a sine qua non of their doctrine. This is not true of other systems of yoga, some of which are avowedly atheistic.

On the purely physical side, the texts say that the aspirant must not be deformed, crippled, weak, blind, deaf, dirty, diseased or paralyzed.

Maithuna or conjugal union then, comes only after a proper period of preparation and proof of competency. The Eastern guru instructs and tests the neophyte for a specific time (usually a year) before actual initiation.

If he proves unsuitable for the Kaula techniques, he will be trained in other disciplines.

Sometimes, students (especially the younger ones) pass all their tests except the final one—that of *maithuna*. In this connection, the writer recalls a somewhat amusing incident that occurred during his residence in India.

It had come to my attention that a certain Tantrik guru in the city of Brindaban was conducting a kind of night school for several boys who aspired to initiation by the Vira ritual—that is, by the Panchatattva, including sexual union.

Armed with a lengthy introduction from my own guru, I traveled to Brindaban with the idea of interviewing the guru there, and perhaps of attending some of his classes. I wished to see how well Tantrik disciplines would lend themselves to group instruction.

Alas, when I arrived, the "school" had been closed. Somewhat sadly, the guru told me why.

"From the last year or more," he said, "I am working strongly to bring the light of the Shastra to each *shishya* (disciple). So, less than a fortnight past, I have arranged a chakra (ritual circle with women) for final *diksha* (initiation).

"All went well, I can tell you, until maithuna. As you may know, the necessary thing in this practice is *jiten-driya*—control of the senses, especially control of the seed or semen. Emission is not allowed for any reason.

"But one of the boys—a Pashu infected with the taint of the Kali Age, did not restrain his bindu as I have taught him. Instead, he is spending his seed, like one devoid of all dharma. Shiva! Shiva! Even a worse thing. To the others of the circle, he is saying, 'This is **very** jolly. Let us indulge.'

"Is there need for saying more? They all were discharging with shouts like players at a polo match or a gymkhana. So the fruit of their long *sadhana* was lost. It is still lost. Now they must find some other path to liberation."

There is little doubt that the concrete rituals, including those that require wine and women, set forth in the original Tantrik scriptures, were meant to be taken literally. Indeed, the stated purpose of the Shastra was to provide the spiritual dwarfs of the Kali age with a ready means of sublimating his animal tendencies.

But Tantrism's rejection of asceticism and of the priestly hierarchy as well as of the caste system, brought it under heavy attack from conservative religious leaders, especially in India.

Exploiting the widespread popular disapproval of meat-eating, wine-drinking, and sexual freedom, enemies of Tantrik rites concentrated their assault upon these three tattvas.

Like the sage Vashishtha before them, they cried, "These are practices contrary to the Vedas!"

As a matter of fact, in early Vedic times, the virile Indo-Aryans who were responsible for Indian civilization at its highest level, were meat-eaters and wine-drinkers.

The famous Indian epic, Ramayana, devotes considerable space to the bibulous and erotic revels of its hero, the pious Brahmin, Rama. Both he and his companions were fond of intoxicants, particularly the alcoholic beverage *sura* (Ram. II, 91.1), which is so roundly damned in the writings of later renunciants.

At one of the forest picnics (Ram. I, 222.14), the scene

described is hardly one to gladden the heart of an anchorite:

"And all did make merry after their desire. And the broad-hipped women, with enticing, swelling breasts and lovely eyes, did besport themselves about with drunken, stumbling gait. Some of the lovelier ones, belonging to Krishna and Arjuna, sported in the forest, and others in the water, and some in the houses, as their pleasure dictated.

"Draupadi and Subhadra, both merry with drink, bestowed clothing and ornaments upon the women. Some danced in wanton abandon, others shrieked and screamed with joy; some amongst the glorious women were laughing, and others drinking the best of *asava*."

Abstinence was enjoined for the Brahmins or priests, as it is today amongst most Protestant Christian denominations.

But as time went on, the prohibition originally laid only upon the Brahmins, was extended to all Hindu society. Drinking and meat-eating, referred to in the literature, came to be interpreted symbolically rather than literally.

(Similarly, in the West, despite the indisputable fact that from his first miracle to his Last Supper, Jesus approved of and drank wine, most Protestant bodies celebrate Holy Communion with unfermented grape juice. They translate the word "wine" in the Gospels as "fruit of the vine.")

Under the relentless pressure of conservative attacks, many Shakta schools began to offer new and more acceptable interpretations of their scriptures.

In this way, Tantrism came eventually to embody three distinct theories of practice. Reactionary opinion described the three theories as corresponding to the three Vedic states of existence—sattva, rajah, and tamas.

Thus, the school claiming to be of the sattvic level, or highest quality, employed symbols rather than actual elements in their practice of Shakta ritual. The so-called Five M's or Five True Things, they asserted, were not to be taken literally.

Instead, wine (*madya*) became merely a term symbolising "the intoxicating knowledge of God." Meat (*mamsha*) really means the tongue (*ma*) used in proper speech (*amsha*). Fish (*matsya*) represents the two vital currents moving in the ida and pingala channels on each side of the spine. When the scriptures refer to sexual union (*maithuna*) they thus indicate meditation upon the primal act of creation. Some texts, in fact, have changed the word from *maithuna* (coition) to *samhita* (union), to indicate union with Brahman.

Those who embraced the second or so-called rajasic sadhana, used material substitutes for the five true things. Instead of wine, they drink coconut juice. Ginger replaces meat. Radish or a plant called *paniphala* is used in lieu of fish. Two flowers, one resembling the male phallus and the other the female yoni, are substituted for maithuna or actual sex union.

The Kaula schools, of course, insist upon a literal interpretation of the texts. They assert that *sadhana* in its symbolical and substitutional forms is fruitless. They point out that the whole principle of Tantrik disciplines is not to shrink from the senses but to conquer them through experience.

Sattvic and rajasic techniques, they maintain, were suitable for preceding and higher ages, but are not practicable for present-day aspirants. They re-emphasize that there is a basic difference between Tantrism and the yoga of asceticism. The path of Tantra is one which develops feeling to the utmost, rather than one aimed at gradually snuffing out the senses. "Perfection can be attained easily by satisfying all desires." [3]

But always for the Tantrik sadhaka there is the warning that, though easy, his way is fraught with many dangers. His method is "risky as handling a snake." One must not venture upon the way of Shaktism without adequate preparation and counsel.

Such counsel, or private instruction, is not easily available, even in India and Tibet. It is commonplace knowledge in both countries today that for every thousand men and women who proclaim themselves gurus, perhaps one genuine initiator may be found.

For the Tantrik aspirant, there are special qualifications to be looked for in a guru. Unlike the chela who plans to follow a path of austerities, and therefore seeks initiation from a renunciate, the Tantrik is urged to choose a married person—man or woman—as his preceptor. The reasons for this are obvious. The grihi or householder is still in and of the world—that "seat of liberation" for the Tantrik disciple.

Intensification of the senses

The traditional yogi who, nominally at least, has renounced the world and who practices techniques aimed

[3] Guhya-samaj Tantra.

at extinguishing desire, is hardly a likely candidate to teach a methodology whose objective is intensification of sense. Thus, the Ganesha Vimarshini clearly states:

"Initiation by an ascetic, by the father, by one living in a forest, or when taken from a renunciant, does no good to a disciple."

The Yogini Tantra also says that initiation should not be taken from one's father. It further states that a student should not be initiated by his or her maternal grandfather, brother, or by one who is younger.

But what of the West, where there are no Tantrik gurus, good or bad?

A Bengali guru, to whom I am indebted for the Westernized form of sadhana included in the present work, had this to say:

"In the Gautamiya Tantra, it is said: 'All two-footed beings in this world, from Brahmin to the lowest, are competent for Kulachara'—that is, for Tantrik initiation.

"This clearly includes the people of your country as well as those of mine. Many here will say, 'But how can there be initiation when there is no guru to give it?'

"To these, my answer is: the supreme Guru is, after all, God. It is only God, acting in and through the consciousness and body of the human guru, who communicates the divine shakti to the disciple. That is the meaning of the passage in Kamakhya Tantra, which says: 'The guru is Shiva Himself.' Likewise in Rudrayamala: 'Shiva alone is guru.'

"Shastra has also made it perfectly clear that the fruits of attainment in previous births are not lost. No matter at what place on earth the Jiva (soul) takes another body, all that he needs to know for his sadhana will, in one way or another, be disclosed to him. This knowledge may come from a dream, a book, a sudden intuition. In the Kularnava Tantra we are even told that Supreme Shiva himself takes human form and secretly wanders about the world in order to assist shishyas (aspirants).

"It is true that much of the Tantrik Shastra must remain veiled or hidden from the Western disciple because of sandha-bhasa. Sandha-bhasa means 'secret word' or so-called 'intentional language.' That is to say, the words of the scriptures have hidden meanings different from those expressed literally.

"Only a guru who knows how to destroy language on one plane of consciousness and to recreate it on another, can impart the deeper essence, and thereby open the gate of good fortune to the sadhaka.

"Even so, who is going to say that Paramashiva is not present in the West? Guptasadhana Tantra declares, 'The entire universe is gurumaya.' In the West you have your own sandha-bhasa—a secret language of symbols and formulae. With it, your men of science have unlocked a potent form of shakti. But to us, unfortunately, it seems the destructive or bhairava aspect of nature. These science gurus have penetrated the cosmic muladhara which lies at the root of creation and have released the coiled and dangerous serpent which now rushes upon us, uncontrolled.

"Who will now save us from this ravage of Durga? Perhaps the present kalpa is nearing an end. Perhaps the hour of final dissolution strikes, when all will return to the fathomless womb of Shakti."

"The art of love is the poor man's art, the one
avenue to ecstasy opens to those who lack all other
talents."

—*Walter Kaufman*

9. *The secret ritual*

As practiced in Tibet and India, the Panchatattva or
Secret Ritual includes some features not easily adaptable
to Western life.

To begin with, there is the question of the shakti or
ceremonial sex partner. In the West, both law and social
usage require that the disciple's ritual consort be his
own wife. If the latter is unwilling or unable to perform
the rite, he is left the alternatives of employing symbolical substitutes or of seeking an illicit union.

Most Eastern gurus carefully select the mudra or
partner to be used in the discipline, the selection being

based upon certain qualities believed to be essential for a successful sadhana.

In most cases, the disciple's wife is found to be satisfactory and is instructed in the ritual according to the guru's individual methods.

Sometimes, however, when a disciple has no wife or when she is not competent for the techniques, a guru may select a parakiya (some other woman), or a sadharani (one who is common or who is paid for her services).

In the latter two instances, the mudra is ritually married to the disciple for the sole purpose of the rite. This ritual wedding is known as a Shiva marriage. It may be terminated at the end of the sadhana, or it may be consecrated as a lifelong spiritual union.

The latter practice brings to mind the "agape" or spiritual love that became an important institution in early Christianity. Tertullian sanctioned such ties for men who craved the companionship of women. In order not to subject the weakness of the flesh to too severe a test, however, he counseled male followers to select as their consorts "the least dangerous among women—widows beautified by faith, endowed with poverty, and sealed by age."

Monks and nuns of the early Church are known to have entered into spiritual espousals of this kind. In some instances, the couple retired to the solitude of the desert, mountains or woods, where the man devoted his life wholly to meditation and prayer, cared for and—it is said—chastely loved by his Platonic helpmate.

In the case of Tantrism, sexual relations with the mudra to whom the disciple has been wed by Shiva nuptials is strictly forbidden outside the sadhana.

The divine union

To understand this point of view, the reader must recall that during maithuna or sacramental union, Tantriks believe that the partners become for the time being a divine couple. Through them flows the cosmic, creative energy of the universe. The mudra is no longer a woman —she is Parashakti herself. The man, likewise, is no longer merely a man, but incarnates Shiva.

Unless this spiritual transformation occurs, Shastra warns that the union is a secular act, therefore carnal and sinful.

On the other hand, when a mystical union of Shiva and Shakti takes place, the sadhaka drinks the ambrosial soma drink, and thereby acquires "the dark moon powers of Shakti."

Successful sadhana, therefore, requires the intelligent participation of both partners. Here in the West, where the guru must of necessity be "the Lord Shiva himself," instruction of a ritual consort not familiar with the rite is limited to literature.

Secret ritual adapted to Western requirements

The secret ritual which follows is one adapted to Western requirements by a Tantrik guru of Bengal who, in addition to expounding the Shastra, has a successful law practice in Calcutta. To preserve his anonymity, we shall call him Pundit Ramkishore Chatterjee, although that is not his real name.

"Some of the more elaborate refinements of sadhana," he explained, "considered virtually indispensable here, have been omitted or abbreviated for non-Indian shishyas.

"For example, it would be most impractical for a student in America to construct a mandala (mystic diagram) with vermilion or red sandal-wood paste, as we do here in India. Nor would it be fruitful for him to do so, without being able to enter it, so to speak, and to meet the forces of the unconscious that would await him there.

"The various mantras given at initiation when a guru is present, also have been omitted. They can not be properly learned or recited from a book.

"I'm well aware," he continued, "that many persons versed in Kuladharma will argue that sadhana without these elements cannot bear fruit. I must insist that it can and that it does. They are but instruments and symbols, and their power is derived from the mind. The mind, therefore, may draw from other sources, by other means.

"During the past twelve years, I have initiated five non-Indians—three Americans and two Europeans. In each instance, the diksha (initiation) was modified to meet their personal requirements and their national backgrounds. In each instance, the yoga was successful."

FOURTH DISCIPLINE

The first two things to be considered in the performance of this discipline are time and place.

As regards the appointed hours, preference is given the period between 7 p.m. and midnight, although the sadhana may be undertaken at any time convenient.

Strict Hindu tradition recognizes only one day each month when the performance of ritual coition is ritu or proper. That is the fifth day following cessation of the shakti's menstrual period. In parts of Tibet and China, this stricture is not observed.

The entire rite should be carried out in dim light, but never in total darkness. The best kind of illumination is a lamp which will produce a deep violet hue. At the time of actual maithuna, this lamp should be placed in a position allowing its rays to fall directly upon the muladhara region of the shakti (female partner).

The room where the sadhana is to take place should be clean, tidy, and well-ventilated. The temperature must be of a level to permit the ritual partners comfortably to remain nude during much of the procedure.

A vase of bright flowers—especially a bouquet of scarlet hibiscus or of red roses—adds a festive touch, but is not essential to the ritual.

The kula-dravya (articles used in the sadhana) are brought into the room at the time the rite is to begin; and the relicts are removed immediately after it is concluded.

These articles are:

A silver tray or china platter upon which have been placed small portions of any freshly cooked meat; fish; cereal biscuits (any commercial brand) or cooked rice; several whole cardamon seeds.

Two glass tumblers and a pitcher of drinking water, to which a few drops of rose water have been added.

A decanter of any kind of wine—sweet or dry.

(Instead of wine, Western students may use brandy, whisky, or liqueur. However, these should be consumed in modest amounts.)

Two liqueur glasses or small cups.

Two candles in holders.

Essence of musk or patchouli.

These materials and instruments should be arranged in an esthetically pleasing way, as one lays a table for a banquet, using a clean linen cloth.

Each article of the festive spread has a symbolical meaning for the sadhaka, According to Shastra, they, together with maithuna, represent the entire universe (jagat-brahmanda).

Wine, says the Mahanirvana Tantra, represents the element fire. It signifies prakriti or creative cosmic energy, which brings joy to man and dispels his sorrows.

In this connexion, psychologists have long been aware of the effect of moderate amounts of wine as a means of unlocking the door to the unconscious mind.

William James, in his "Varieties of Religious Experience," notes that: "The sway of alcohol over mankind is due to its power to stimulate the mystical faculties of human nature, usually crushed to earth by the cold fact and dry criticisms of the sober hour . . . It brings him from the chill periphery of things to the radiant core . . . It makes him for the moment one with truth."

But just as Tantrik scriptures warn against excess, so James observes:

"It is part of the deeper mystery and tragedy of life that whiffs and gleams of something that we immediately recognize as excellent, should be vouchsafed to so many of us only in the fleeting early phases of what in its totality is so degrading a poisoning."

Meat, the second tattva, which stimulates growth of the body and development of the mind, signifies the element air. It also represents all animal life upon the earth.

Fish, related symbolically to the element water, stands for the generative powers of the body and the flow of prana through the three principal nadis. With it, the sadhaka identifies himself with aquatic forms of life.

Parched cereal unites one with all vegetable life, and through it, with those geodetic currents drawn from the soil as the nourishment of terrestrial life. The cereal embodies, so to speak, the element earth.

Similarly, as explained earlier in the present work, the cardamom seeds illustrate the bifold structure of physical creation, wrapped in its sheath (kosha) of maya or veiling. Mystics of all faiths have affirmed this duality in every aspect of life, pointing to it as the source of all creative activity.

Finally, the fifth tattva or sexual union, is ether, the basic substratum behind all creation—the very root of the visible world.

So the maithuna couple, if they persevere in their embrace, come to feel and know the supreme bliss that permeates the process of creation. Even the non-Tantrik scriptures of India note the sacramental nature of the act. Hence the passage in the celebrated Brihad-aranyaka Upanishad, which Edward Carpenter—ignorant of its inner meaning—called "obscene":

"Her lower part is the sacrificial altar: her hairs the sacrificial grass, her skin the soma-press. The two labia of the vulva are the fire in the middle. Verily, as great as is the world of him who performs the Vajapeya sacrifice, so great is the world of him who, knowing this, practices sexual intercourse; he turns the good deeds of the woman to himself; but he, who without knowing this, practices sexual intercourse, his good deeds women turn to themselves." [1]

Immediately prior to the sadhana, both partners are instructed to bathe carefully, from head to toe. In addition to purely esthetic considerations, the bath is de rigueur in the Tantrik ritual because bio-electrical currents must flow freely between the couple during bodily contact required in later phases of the sadhana. Experiments have shown that these currents attain their greatest intensity in the genital area of the human body.

Upon emerging from the bath, the shakti anoints herself liberally with her favorite scent (more than used for street wear), provided it is one of the better French perfumes, most of which include in their formula, either musk or civet.

She then dons a negligee of thin silk, nylon or fine linen. Orthodox Tantrik opinion holds that this garment should be red, or a shade close to that of the hibiscus or China rose, which is the symbolic flower of Tantrism.

The sadhaka wears a dressing gown or robe of any material such as linen or silk, provided it is a non-conductor. It may be of any color or design.

If both ritual partners have practiced the preliminary disciplines (as detailed in the foregoing portions of this book) they enter the sadhana chamber together, and both proceed with the first step of the secret ritual, the yoni mudra.

If the shakti has not undergone the preparatory train-

1 Brihad-aranyaka Upanishad (Radhakrishnan trans.) VI. 4.3.

ing, the male shisshya enters the room alone and calls his mudra (partner) after he has completed the initial discipline, which follows:

After lighting the candles, he seats himself in the practice posture he has found to be most suitable for meditation. After emptying the residual air from the lungs, he equalizes the breath and brings it under control by pranayama (inhale seven, hold one, exhale seven; repeat twelve times).

Upon inhaling to begin the thirteenth breath cycle, he holds his breath for seven counts before exhaling to the count of seven. During the period of retention, he focuses his awareness strongly upon the muladhara center, situated between the anus and the root of the genitals.

As he holds his breath, he stimulates this center by contracting the sphincter muscles of the anus. Meanwhile, he visualizes creative union taking place between Shiva and Shakti; that is, between cosmic consciousness (purusha) and cosmic energy (prakriti). As this union occurs, he imagines a vital current flowing upward through the central channel (sushumna) of his spine and on to the top of his head.

This retention cycle is repeated twelve times. Then the mudra is called in and the rite proceeds, with both partners participating.

At the table-altar, the shakti sits on the sadhaka's left hand. When both are seated, and after a moment's silence, the sadhaka performs the ceremony known as the panchikarana, thus:

With the index finger of his right hand, he taps the wine decanter, exclaiming "Phat!"

Then, while uttering the seed syllable, "Hung," he

makes a gesture as though veiling the decanter. This done, he sits back and regards the wine for a moment with unblinking gaze. Thereafter, he joins the thumb and ring finger of his left hand and gestures toward the decanter, saying: "namah."

Finally, removing the stopper, he grasps the decanter in his left hand. Closing his right nostril with his right hand, he brings the wine close to the ida or left nostril and inhales the aroma from the vintage.

Turning his head away from the decanter, he exhales through the pingala or right nostril. This smelling procedure is repeated three times. It is done for the purpose of purifying the three nadis or subtle channels of psychic energy.

Thereafter, he intones the following mantra:

"Devata bhava siddhaye."

The two small glasses or cups are filled two-thirds full of wine. One is passed to the shakti, and the ritual partners lift their glasses in unison and drain the contents.

Thereupon, the sadhaka refills them, again only two-thirds full. Then the couple each takes a small piece of meat from the plate, holding it between the thumb and third finger of the right hand. They mentally repeat the words, Shiva, Shakti, Sadha-Shiva, Ishvara, Vidya, Kala.

Realizing that they are in the presence of the Devi, they reflect: "I purify my gross body with atma-tattva." Then each consumes the piece of meat.

This is followed by wine, the glass or cup being held between the thumb and third finger of the left hand.

The sadhaka refills the wine glasses.

Now a small portion of fish is taken in the same manner as the meat. Holding it, the partners mentally recite the Mulamantra: Deva bhava siddhaye. The wine is consumed.

After the sadhaka has again refilled the glasses, the same karana is repeated, using the parched grain or biscuit. Once more the glasses are drained and refilled.

At this point, a portion of each of the shuddhi (meat, fish, and biscuit) is eaten, followed with wine.

"Then let them each take up his own cup and meditate upon the kula-kundalini as being divine consciousness in the body, and who is spread from the root chakra to the tip of the tongue. . . ." [2]

The worshippers again empty their glasses, which are then filled with water. This is used to rinse the mouth thoroughly.

From the shuddhi-patra (plate or platter holding ritual food), the sadhaka takes a cardamom and passes it to his shakti, who receives it in the palm of her left hand. He then takes one for himself. Both partners break open the outer sheath or husk. Regarding the bivalvular grain within—two halves forming a unity within the enfolding sheath—they recall that all creation is likewise a unity, which appears to be a duality when viewed through the veil of prakriti. They reflect that this duality constitutes a polarity and that the same polarity is present within them.

Then the cardamoms are removed and chewed to sweeten the breath.

Thereafter, the partners leave the table and repair to a couch or bed, where the maithuna is to take place.

The shakti now disrobes (except for any jewels she may wish to wear) and seats herself upright on the edge

[2] Mahanirvana Tantra: VI. 191–193.

of the bed or couch. The sadhaka stands before her.

The violet lamp is lighted and placed in such a position that its light falls upon the nude body of the shakti.

Viewing her now as an incarnation of the Sapphire Devi, the sadhaka gazes upon her with admiration and awe, as one pondering the mystery of creation and the unfathomable secret of being. For she is "extremely subtle; the awakener of pure knowledge, the embodiment of all bliss."

Again, the sadhaka contemplates her as "the unsullied treasure house of beauty, the shining protoplast, the begetter of all that is, that inscrutably becomes, dies and is born again."

In the Lalita Vistara it is written that she it is "whose slender waist, bending beneath the burden of her breasts' ripe fruit, swells into jewelled hips, heavy with the promise of infinite maternities."

Unless the sadhaka can thus envision his shakti, he is counselled to proceed no further with the sadhana. For, according to virtually all Tantrik opinion, without such realization, the maithuna which follows is a carnal and secular act, no different from ordinary sexual intercourse.

After observing the shakti in this way, the sadhaka places his hand over his heart and recites the mantram: "Shiva hum, So' hum," which means, "I am Shiva; I am She." He thereby identifies himself with the cosmic union of Shiva-Shakti.

Then he projects into his shakti's body the life of the Devi by a rite referred to in Tantrik texts as nyasa. The word is derived from a Sanskrit root meaning "to place," and the modus operandi consists in placing the tips of the fingers on certain parts of the shakti's body, uttering the appropriate mantra. The purpose of this practice is to awaken vital forces that lie dormant in these regions of the gross body.

Using the index and middle fingers of his right hand, the sadhaka lightly and deliberately touches the shakti's heart area, crown of her head, three eyes (that is, center of forehead and two eyelids); hollow of the throat, left and right ear lobes, breasts, upper arms (left and right), navel, thighs, knees, feet, and yoni.

As he executes these motions, he recites the following mantra, either mentally or aloud:

"Hling . . . kling . . . kandarpa . . . svaha."

The sadhaka next removes his own robe, and the partners lie together upon the bed, the shakti on the left of the sadhaka. She reclines flat on her back, and he upon his *left* side, facing her.

In the event that the sadhaka's breath flow is not already through the pingala or right side, it will soon take that channel, after he has lain for a short time on his left side.

When he clearly perceives that the flow is through the pingala, he is ready to assume the maithuna position, which is accomplished in this way:

The shakti raises both her legs by bending her knees and pulling them upward toward her chest. The sadhaka then swings the upper portion of his body away from hers and brings his lingam into close contact with her yoni. She then lowers her legs, and he places his right leg between her legs. Properly carried out, the maneuvers bring the sex organs of the ritual partners into close contact, which may be prolonged over a period of time without tension or discomfort.

Lying thus fully relaxed, the sadhaka gently parts

the labia of the yoni and partially inserts his lingam. Deep penetration of the vagina at this point is neither necessary nor desirable. But close contact between the lingam and the moist membrane of the inner yoni is important.

The sadhaka and his consort now lie completely motionless and relaxed for a period of thirty-two minutes. During this interval, the co-partners visualize the flow of pranic currents between them, the strongest being at the point of contact between the sexual organs. Such concentration is not forced or tense, but performed in a detached, almost somnolent way.

Gradually each partner will become aware of a rising tide of pleasurable sensation, growing in intensity as psychic energy courses through the reproductive organs and the chakras.

According to Pandit Chatterjee, among Western students practicing the sadhana, a sudden acme of sensation occurs at some point between the twenty-eighth and thirty-second minute of practice. This abrupt excitation, unlike anything ever experienced before, results in orgastic and involuntary contraction of the body's total musculature.

A clearly-perceived decrease of tension follows, as the direction of the pranic currents is reversed, now flowing inward rather than outward, entering the nadis of the subtle body and energizing the entire organism.

This inexpressible experience of unity is called samarasa in the Tantrik texts; that is, a state which is nirvanic. That is why maithuna has such an important place in Tantrik disciplines. By means of this inversion, this flowing back of pranic currents, reabsorption of the cosmos occurs. Time and eternity become one, Shiva and Shakti are wed within the sadhaka's own being, and he knows the totalization that preceded creation of the universe.

Unless this inflowing of energy occurs, together with the rapturous state just described, the sadhana has failed and ought to be repeated again at a later date.

In their instruction of the sadhaka, Tantrik gurus lay great emphasis upon cautioning against allowing ejaculation to occur. Such a hard and fast rule obviously calls for great self-control and previous training on the part of the male partner in the sadhana. At the same time, it places Tantrik sadhana beyond the reach of the libertine, the voluptuary, and the idly curious.

If, during maithuna, the sadhaka feels ejaculation to be imminent, he is instructed to prevent it by holding his breath, at the same time turning his tongue backward as far as he can against the roof of his mouth.

In India and Tibet, yogis gradually lengthen their tongues by certain practices until they can reverse them, turning them backward into the hollow space beneath the epiglottis.

For the Western aspirant, however, it is sufficient merely to curl the tongue backward as far as possible, suspend the breath, and contract the anal muscles as in practicing the discipline which preceded maithuna.

It is important to bear in mind that the immediate aim is the temporary and simultaneous arrest of breath, thought, and semen. The Goraksha Samhita declares:

"So long as the breath is in motion, the semen moves also. When breath ceases to move, the semen is likewise at rest."

If involuntary emission does occur, then the sadhana is terminated, since it will then bear no fruit. At the same time, gurus tell their students that if ejaculation is unintentional, it ought not to discourage further attempts to practice the rite.

If the sadhaka is successful in overcoming the urge to indulge in conventional orgasm, he continues to maintain his maithuna position for several minutes following the samarasa state. This time may gradually be extended to two or three hours, if the couple mutually desires it.

The ritual may be terminated in either of two ways:

(1) The sadhaka withdraws and "returns once more to the tavern"; that is, he repeats the yoni mudra technique with which the sadhana began.

(2) Fully relaxed in body and mind, and soothed by the rapture of true union, the couple's samarasa state passes into normal slumber. Both then awaken deeply refreshed and more harmonious in their everyday relations with each other.

Pundit Chatterjee recalled two instances in which marital alliances, torn by emotional conflicts, were restored to harmony and mutual love by the practice of Tantrik maithuna.

It should be emphasized that the sadhana just outlined is a yogic discipline and rite. It is not related in any way to conventional sexual intercourse. As a Tantrik ritual, it is properly performed only once during a lunar month—that on the shakti's day or the fifth day following cessation of the menses.

Even so, some of its features may profitably be adapted to ordinary intercourse, if the couple wishes to do so.

For example, in the secular act, the period of immobility may be observed, followed by actual orgasm.

There is little doubt that many wives in the West—where a brief and sometimes overly abrupt union leaves them tense and dissatisfied—would welcome a more deliberate approach to the sexual experience.

The need for greater concentration and mental awareness during coition is another Tantrik practice that could be adopted with beneficial results in the West. It should be noted that this implies not only the awareness of physical sensations, but also feelings of love, devotion and tenderness towards one's co-partner in the act.

Dr. Wilhelm Reich, a tireless researcher in biology and natural science, observed that well-adjusted individuals never talk or laugh during the sexual act, unless it be with words of tenderness. He points out that both talking and laughing indicate a serious lack of the capacity for surrender. For the latter requires the individual's undivided absorption in the sensations of samarasa.

Dr. Reich stated unequivocally that men to whom such surrender means being "feminine" are always emotionally disturbed.

As previously stated, the secret ritual of Tantrism has higher aims, however, than merely improving sexual relations between man and wife.

According to Tantra, the priceless gifts of maithuna are wisdom and moksha (liberation from material bondage).

The ancient teachings remind us again and again that through this ritual, the jivatma or individual self, transcends time and death, to share in the immortal being of the Paratma or divine self.

Thus the mind of the sadhaka is no longer confined within the limits of logic and conscious reason. Floating free, so to speak, he gives himself over to the strange impulses and intuitive knowledge that come to him out of the unknown.

He enters the secret background of nature, the world of the artist and the saint. He is like the swan that the poet Rilke describes, who, after walking awkwardly upon the earth, enters the water—"soft against his breast, which now how easily together flows behind him in a little wake of waves . . . while he, infinitely silent, self-possessed, and ever more mature, is pleased to move serenely on his majestic way."

In our day, when man's rational faculty, which has transformed our lives, has also provided the immediate means of destroying them, there is an urgent need for this voyage of the soul.

Rationalist critics may dismiss such a mystical projection as a form of escapism. But does such an opinion have any real foundation beyond the materialist's desire to consider all supralogical experiences as clinical data?

Rather, ought we not to ask ourselves whether the kind of reality to be experienced through Tantrik maithuna is not preferable to the concept whose ultimate meaning is summed up in such terms as "over-kill," "acceptable level of risk," and "first-strike capacity?"

Surely, Tantrik sadhana moves toward a more satisfying plane of existence; one in which there is more love and, in a final sense, more stability.

> "Pierced at a distance by the thorn of *sanyama*, the virgin yields her essence which, like moonlight, soothes those burned by the three-tongued flame of misery."
>
> —*Fragment of a Lost Tantra*

10. *The subtle embrace*

It is a common boast among Tantriks of certain Kaula sects that they enjoy the desired fruit of *maithuna* without any physical contact with the woman.

Conversely, a female initiate may effect the same kind of subtle union with a virile young male, as we have noted in the instance of the Ka'a sect of Tibetan nuns, who use the energy so derived for healing and magical rites.

The various disciplines for accomplishing this end differ with the several sects that practice them, but all are based upon the principle of bioelectrical duality common to most Tantras.

As previously explained in the chapter on sound, all breathing creatures unconsciously utter an involuntary mantram—"hang-sah, hang-sah,"—made by the incoming and outflowing breath. Known as the *ajapa mantra,* it corresponds to the cosmic pulse, the breath of God, in a manner of speaking.

The divine rhythm

Vital functions of living organisms follow this pranic pattern, manifesting themselves rhythmically by expansion and contraction.

Even in the single-celled amoeba, this pulsation is to be found in motion of the vacuoles.

In higher forms of life, including man, the divine rhythm moves constantly through the various organs, providing the dynamic that makes them function.

The heart has its systole and diastole; the intestines their alternating motion called peristalsis; the muscles, striped and smooth, have respectively contractive and serpentine movements.

Governing all these rhythms of the body are electrical processes, known to Western science as "pacemakers."

Tantriks, of course, regard all bioelectricity as modes of Shakti, the primal energy. They assert that opposite polarities generate constant motion in both physical and subtle bodies, as energy passes from centers of higher potential to those of lower potential.

At the time of puberty and for several years thereafter, a natural stirring of the serpent power or *kundalini* occurs. Although it vitalizes all the chakras of the
subtle body, it is most potently concentrated in the
genitals, whence it is discharged to some extent into the
young person's aura.

Poltergeist Phenomena

It is interesting to note that Western investigators are
beginning to suspect what Tantriks have taught for centuries—that psycho-sexual energy generated in this way
can produce startling and inexplicable phenomena in
the physical world.

One of the chief sources of data available to our in-
quirers is that of poltergeist phenomena.

Poltergeists are the "noisy ghosts" assumed to be responsible for various kinds of unexplained disturbances.
These include loud knockings and terrifying sounds;
mysterious levitation of articles, which fly through the
air or move about a room; and the sudden appearance of
intense heat on walls and bedsteads.

Significantly, the poltergeist or "rattling spirit" has
never been confined to one locality or age. Rather, he is
known in all areas of our globe, both savage and civi-
lized. Recorded accounts of his strange behaviour date
back as far as 856 B.C.

In centuries of observation and study of poltergeist
mischief, researchers have all agreed that one factor
seems always to be present at the scene of the enigmatic
outbreaks. The baffling incidents occur in the immedi-

ate vicinity of young women, or in less frequent in-stances, of boys near the age of puberty.

Harry Price, the noted investigator of psychic phe-nomena, observed that in 95% of the poltergeist cases studied by him, a young girl was closely associated with the strange disturbances. In the remaining 5%, a young boy seemed to have some connection with it.

He further remarks upon the fact that puberty, ado-lescence and sexual excitement or trauma very often mark the onset or the termination of poltergeist phe-nomena. He cites an instance in which the paranormal events associated with a young girl disappeared over-night with her first menstruation.

He also calls attention to the fact that during experi-ments conducted in Vienna, a subject who had the ability to make objects move at a distance (a power known as psycho-kinesis), displayed greater energy when a sympathetic young woman acted as control.

From the Tantrik point of view, the incendiary effects of poltergeist activity are also highly significant in point-ing to the source of the energy at work. The prime attri-bute of kundalini energy is heat.

A typical case of poltergeist heat phenomena was re-ported from Cidevelle Abbey in France. Among the curious incidents were heavy rumblings and blows on the walls of a room. Some person evidently schooled in matters of the occult suggested to the Curé that iron spikes be driven into the walls. When this was done, smoke and flames issued from the holes made by them. The extraordinary happenings ceased when two boys, aged twelve and fourteen, who occupied the room, were removed from the Abbey.

A similar instance in which intense heat was produced

in conjunction with other poltergeist phenomena, was reported by the Rev. L. A. Foyster, who resided in the celebrated Borley Rectory in Essex, an edifice known as "the most haunted house in England."

The rector noted in his diary that whilst he was entertaining some visitors one day, a mysterious fire broke out in an unused bedroom. When he entered the room, he found one portion of a wall incandescent, glowing like an ember.

This and subsequent disturbances of a weird nature finally forced the clergyman and his family to vacate the rectory. It was later occupied by Price and a number of associates who wished to study the phenomena at close range.

In 1938, a message was received by automatic writing, stating that the haunted rectory would be destroyed by fire.

A year later, the prophecy came true. It burned to the ground mysteriously one midnight. Spectators at the scene insisted that they had seen phantoms amid the leaping flames.

When the charred ruins were completely cleared in 1945, in one of the cellars workmen found human bones that were identified as those of a young woman.

Tantriks say that the circumstances and nature of such phenomena associated with poltergeists strongly suggest that the energy manifested in them is sexual in origin.

A number of contemporary investigators in the West tend to agree. One of them, Dr. Hereward Carrington, after studying many occurrences of the kind, advanced the view that libido was indeed the secret dynamo providing energy for the phenomena.

In his book, "The Story of Psychic Science," he notes that the peculiar kind of energy witnessed in these proceedings seems to be radiated from the body of the human agent just at the time sexual vigor is blossoming into maturity.

"It would almost seem," he writes, "as though these energies, instead of taking their normal course, were somehow turned to another channel at such times and were externalized beyond the limits of the body, producing the manifestations in question."

Dr. John Layard, a Jungian psychologist, sees in poltergeist disturbances indications of a deep and unresolved conflict in the personality of the human agent responsible for them. He enunciates the principle in terms of polarity, and his statement sounds as though he were quoting from one of the Tantras.

He says there exists, a priori, in such a personality situations of extreme tension, "when the two poles of the personality are trying to join, but cannot."

While adolescence is the classic time for extraordinary display of psycho-sexual energy, the same energy is sometimes discharged into the surrounding ether by adults during sexual excitation.

For example, the husband of an Austrian sensitive reported that during the acme of sexual embrace with his wife, small ornaments on the mantel would move about mysteriously.

In the flow of such energy from one person to another, the current or radiation will move toward the weaker of the two. It thus behaves in the same way as electrical energy.

As regards the latter, it is well known that if a highly charged body is connected to one of lower potential, current flows from the stronger to the weaker, until equalization between the two charges occurs.

As a matter of fact, the theory has long been held throughout the world that a person of advanced age who lives in prolonged and intimate contact with youth, apparently draws vitality and health from the younger person or persons. This is all the more true if the younger is of the opposite sex and in glowing good health.

It was no doubt this knowledge which prompted the retainers of ailing King David of antiquity to search his kingdom for a young girl who might help restore his waning physical strength.

"Now King David was old and stricken in years," the scripture relates, "and they covered him with clothes, but he gat no heat. Wherefore his servants said unto him, Let there be sought for my Lord the king a young virgin: and let her stand before the king, and let her cherish him, and let her lie in his bosom, that my Lord the king may get heat.

"So they sought for a fair damsel throughout all the coasts of Israel, and found Abishag, a Shunnamite, and brought her to the king." [1]

Later, with the rise of the Troubadours in Medieval Europe, the same Tantrik technique makes its appearance once more.

One of the least adequately explored aspects of the Troubadour movement in the feudal courts is the Tantrik origin of its secret disciplines.

The relationship between the true Troubadour and the object of his love (usually the wife of a feudal lord,

[1] I Kings I:1–3.

but sometimes a maid) was more than that of mere patroness and poet.

The Troubadours had a special name for this relationship. They called it *donnoi*. A careful examination of their celebrated love songs will quickly make clear the exact nature of the relationship denoted by that word.

Some speak of a certain manner of gazing at the beloved so as to awaken slumbering forces in the lover. Others describe how they undressed their lady, gazed rapturously at her naked body, made passes over it, and spent hours at a time with her nude form pressed close to their own.

But in no place is there a reference to any kind of marked orgasm or to intercourse in the conventional sense of the word.

On the contrary, they declared that "he knows nothing of *donnoi* who wants to possess his lady carnally."

William of Poitiers, one of the first Troubadours, unequivocally spells out the Tantrik nature of *donnoi*. He says:

"I want to retain my lady in order to refresh my heart and renew my body so well that I cannot age. He will live a hundred years who succeeds in possessing the joy of his love."

Centuries before, a grateful Roman by the name of Hermippus had raised a marble monument to the same formula. The inscription read:

"To Aesculapius and Sanitas this is placed by L. Clodius Hermippus, who lived 115 years and five days by perspiration of a young virgin, causing great wonder to all physicians. May posterity lead similar lives in this fashion."

Parenthetically, it should be borne in mind that in classical usage (as in Biblical and Hindu texts), the word "virgin" did not have exactly the same meaning as that given it in most countries today.

It referred to any unmarried girl past the age of puberty, usually one who enjoyed the vitality and burgeoning beauty of good health.

The term used by the ancients in referring to a girl who had never known sexual intercourse was more explicit: *virgo intacta.*

Mention should be made in the present context also of another Medieval group who apparently held certain views that were unquestionably Tantrik in origin, namely, King Arthur and his knights.

De Rougement, in his "Love in the Western World," quotes Rene Nelli on the erotic magic of the Grail as follows:

"This erotic magic was inspired first of all by a belief that the female body displayed by its mere presence certain supernatural powers, the same that were attributed to the Grail. (The Grail rejuvenated those who contemplated it.)"

Nelli's analysis does not make clear the important fact that the female body referred to was that of a beautiful young virgin, the *kumari* of Tantrik treatises.

Persecution of the Church eventually extirpated such sects as the Troubadours, Cathars and mystic lovers of the Middle Ages, but the ancient belief that in virginity could be found an elixir of life persisted in the West, as it always had in the East.

In the eighteenth century, the wife of a French physician operated a successful establishment in Paris, which offered rejuvenation to old men and renewed vigor to impotent young men. The technique used was close contact with virgins.

Restif de la Bretonne, historian of sexual life in the Paris of his day, describes the procedure in some detail.

He says that girls recruited for the purpose had to be in glowing good health, and in the first bloom of maidenhood. Urban Paris was apparently unable to provide consorts who could meet those requirements. Most of them were found in the rural areas of France.

The Tantrik nature of the practice, despite its low moral character and setting, is evident from the procedure followed. Each girl was carefully inspected for hidden defects and thereafter underwent a period of training by Madame Janus, as the operator of the strange lupanar was called. They had to be of average height, well-formed, of pleasant countenance and disposition; and to walk with the lithe step of a leopard.

The girls—there were forty of them—were placed on a diet which, it was believed, would greatly increase their vitality and bring to full charge the electrical potential in each. They followed a strict regimen of daily physical exercise, personally supervised by Madame Janus herself.

As in the case of Tantrik *maithuna,* both the male client and the two virginal partners who were to serve him, were given perfumed baths, followed by a brisk rubdown to increase circulation and build bioelectricity in the body.

The man then retired for the night, lying between two girls, one a blonde, the other a brunette.

All three slept on the right side, the brunette closely pressed against the man's back and he, in turn, in close contact with the nude back of the blonde.

This course of "treatment" continued nightly for a

little more than three weeks. Each pair of virgins was relieved by two fresh ones after eight days of continuous service.

Madame Janus declared that a girl's restorative powers were exhausted in about a year if she was employed every night, without periods of respite. If, on the other hand, she took two-week intermissions to rest up and to revitalize herself, she would be effective as a rejuvenator for as long as three years.

Mahatma Gandhi and virgin consorts

In our own day, it has been reported that the late Mahatma Gandhi sometimes slept chastely in bed with young girls. The English assumed that he did this to prove his power over temptation, but Tantriks say he found the subtle emanations of virgins a valuable source of energy during his long and debilitating fasts, undertaken in the course of his struggle with the British Raj.

According to Tantrik teachings, during a night-long contact of the kind just described, a polarization takes place which, while not of the all-pervading, plenary character of ritual union, is nonetheless a subtle kind of *maithuna*.

Far more potent, of course, is the discipline performed at a distance and without bodily contact of any kind. An epoptic treatise in the possession of a Kaula sect in Bengal tells how this may be accomplished.

The sadhaka is instructed, first of all, to find a *nayika* or virgin consort suitable for the practice. She may be a stranger casually encountered, who remains unaware that the *sadhana* is being performed. Or she may be a female servant, a pupil, or a girl paid for her service.

But from whatever quarter she comes, she must meet certain requirements as to appearance and physical condition.

In general, these qualifications are the same as those prescribed for the partner in the secret ritual. That is, she must be of good health, possess a body without physical defects, have fully developed breasts (a sine qua non among all Hindus), prominent mons veneris, and lustrous, abundant hair.

In practice, the sadhana is most often performed as an unauthorized intrusion. Without attracting attention, the practicant places himself within the girl's auric range, that is, at a distance of six feet or less.

Making certain that he is unobserved, either by the girl or by others, he then makes *sanyama* on the consort's sex chakra.

Sanyama means bringing the mind to a point and focussing it on an object, mental image or idea. The process embodies three steps.

First, withdrawing the awareness from objects of sense, the yogi strongly visualizes the *muladhara* center, situated midway between the anus and genitals. This may be conceived as a triangle, inside which is a brilliant red, twisted tongue of flame.

For the space of several minutes, his mind dwells solely upon this image, without wavering or "spreading" to related ideas or train of thoughts.

Such one-pointedness is accomplished, not by willing it (or the law of reverse effort will take over and the end result will be opposite that desired), but by the imagination. In a quiet, tranquil, almost detached mood, he turns his attention fully upon the image of the chakra, as though it were before his eyes.

Once a degree of full concentration is established, the yogi, oblivious of all else save his vision of the triangle and its tongue of flame, once more allows his thoughts to move. Only, this time they move around the image he has held in focus.

The effect may be compared with the stopping of a motion picture film during projection. All action is arrested. A single image remains frozen upon the screen, to be studied in detail for as long a period as desired.

Then motion is resumed and the flow of visual continuity goes on. We see not only the object or view that was fixed in the stationary frame, but related features, either of setting or of detail.

So it is with the sadhaka, who now allows the continuity of thoughts to resume. He finds that instead of the promiscuous series of ideas that usually flow through the conscious mind when it is given free rein, a meaningful and associated pattern of mental perceptions emerges.

Unlike ordinary reverie, his present thought is charged with emotion. He not only visualizes the objective of his *sanyama;* he also strongly *feels* it. It becomes a vivid dream of the yoga sleep.

At this point, according to the text, he experiences rapture. That is to say, he forgets his own identity, losing himself in the intuitional contact with the muladhara chakra of the girl before him.

After an interval of mystical unity, which may last for a brief moment or for an hour, he rouses himself to cognitive awareness.

Then noting the girl's respiratory rhythm, as indicated by the rising and falling of the chest, he begins to breathe in unison. As he does so, he stimulates the electrical discharge of his own muladhara by contracting the sphincter muscles of the anus.

If he has properly "locked on," he can now speed up the respiratory rate of his shakti by breathing more rapidly himself.

With a quicker vibration thus established in both sadhaka and sadharani, the yogi visualizes an invisible, but powerful current flowing from the muladhara center of the younger person into his own. As he rhythmically contracts the anal sphincter, he mentally repeats the mantra, "Hang-sah; Hang-sah."

Success of the sadhana is signalled by the rise of body temperature, especially in the region of the genitals. Essentially, the feeling of warmth that begins to emanate from the muladhara is activity of the kundalini, and is related to the *tumo* or psychic heat extensively dealt with in Tibetan texts.

To Western readers, who have inherited the rationalist, materialistic philosophy of their civilization, a procedure such as that just described may appear fantastic or naively imaginative.

They should bear in mind, however, that Tantra is based firmly upon the premise that an exchange of psychic energy is constantly going on between person and person, planet and planet, universe and universe.

The Shastra further holds that *sanyama,* or the practice of combined concentration, meditation and rapture, can arouse slumbering forces within one's own body or in that of others.

By the same technique, these forces can be directed

from one point to another, anywhere in the universe.

The reason is this: mind and matter are but two different modes or polarities of the same supreme Power—the one subtle, the other gross.

It seems clear to the Tantrik that one can act upon the other.

"How long does youth endure?
So long as we are loved."

—*Golden Book of Diana*

11. *The wellspring of youth*

Western students invariably ask: will the practice of Tantrik sadhana help me to stay young? What kind of diet does the Shastra prescribe? Are there disciplines that can be used to cure illness?

Such queries reflect the dominant preoccupation with the physical body that has come to be an outstanding characteristic of occidental civilization.

At no time nor place in history have such care and attention been lavished upon the fleshly form. Never before has youth, per se, been of such paramount importance to a whole population that they would spend enormous amounts of time and money in a desperate attempt to remain young.

It has been reliably estimated that eighty percent of all contemporary men and women in the Western world have no higher aim in life than to live in comfort and safety, and to be admired.

Thanks to tremendous advances in technology and medicine, this ideal has been largely achieved. Only within the most recent years has the threat of nuclear extinction hung monstrously in our blue heaven.

Even the Westerner's religion, Christianity, has joined the popular chorus clamouring for an earthly paradise. Disregarding their Founder's clear-cut declaration—"My kingdom is not of this world"—most Christian denominations today dedicate their time, money and energies to implementing the "social gospel," that is, to the problems of earthly existence and to ways of improving it for all men.

The Tantrik view, on the other hand, while acknowledging the importance of earthly life as an arena for soul experience, insists upon the primacy of the spirit.

Tantra—The fountain of youth

The gross body is given careful attention and care, not as an end in itself, but only because it is an instrument of the soul, to be used for attaining moksha or liberation.

Tantriks claim that their sadhana, more than other systems of yoga, bestows youth upon the aspirant because of its concern with the muladhara or sex chakra. As previously explained, Tantra regards this subtle center as the control station for organic and cellular functions that, in turn, influence the ageing processes of the body.

Research by Western scientists seeking a fountain of youth for material reasons, supports this view.

For example, Dr. Eugen Steinach, the Viennese physiologist noted for his pioneer work in human rejuvenation, noted that senility is directly related to sexuality.

He said that sex is the most obvious key to the process of ageing because the sex glands are what he called the "root of life."

He observed that, just as sexual glands produce physical and psychic maturity, induce and preserve the period of human flowering for shorter or longer periods, depending upon the individual, so also their function is responsible for the fading of the body and the diminishing of vitality, both physical and mental.

This being true, it follows that in the sex chakra we have the means for not only increasing the store of energy available during the early years, but an instrument for its restoration in the period of old age.

The youthfulness, both in appearance and behavior, of most Americans—so striking to people of other countries—is attributable not so much to improved cosmetics and better nutrition as to the constant stimulation of the sex center by advertising, literature, movies, TV, and so on.

Most rejuvenation formulae put forward by metaphysical groups in the United States fail dismally because of two things.

First of all, they encourage their followers to suppress

the sexual function or to deny it full expression. In so doing, they also arrest the flow of life-giving hormones which alone can insure youthful vigor to the organism.

In the second instance, they prescribe a system of meditation that accomplishes a result exactly opposite that desired. This is true because of a principle known as the law of reversed effort.

When we voluntarily focus the attention upon an idea (as in meditation), and will a condition to come about, the negative force of our will immediately appears as a counter-suggestion. The more we concentrate, the stronger our mental effort in the direction of a given goal, the greater the resistance to that effort.

Every alcoholic who has tried to give up drinking by willing himself to do so knows that the more violent his resolve not to touch another drop, the sooner he will find himself with another bottle in his hand.

Similarly, the greater effort you make to stay young, the greater the forces you set in motion to make you older. Perhaps the most potent of these negative forces is fear. The fear of ill health and fear of age produces a kind of poison that hastens both conditions.

No matter what diet you follow, what exercises you take, what vitamins you swallow, if you are old at heart —that is, sexually old—senility will soon follow.

On the other hand, Tantrik gurus worthy of the utmost confidence have asserted repeatedly that youth can be maintained throughout the normal lifespan.

Their prescript is simple: elimination of the corrosive acids that cause formation of the death element in man. These "acids" formed by our reaction to influences outside ourselves, soon make their presence known, first in the quality of our thinking.

The spontaneity, the enthusiasm, the readiness to change—which characterize youth—gradually disappear. Habitual patterns of thought emerge. We become "set in our ways."

Neutralizing the corrosive acids of age

To quicken the vibrations of both body and mind, and thus to neutralize the corrosive acids of age, so to speak, Tantrik sadhana rouses the cosmic energy coiled in the root chakra.

This action releases neurohormones into the bloodstream of the gross body, re-invigorating the physical powers.

The mental faculties are likewise revitalized, creating a more active and seeking inclination in the mind, a dissatisfaction with the status quo.

The over-all guiding principle in Tantrik rejuvenation is, of course, love—that is, reintegration of the two polar streams. And the method, par excellence, for achieving this end is successful maithuna.

Tantrik views on diet

In the matter of diet, with one or two notable exceptions, Tantriks follow the same regimen as that of other yogis and of Hindus in general. Outside the panchatattva ritual, they rarely eat meat or drink alcoholic beverages.

However, their eating habits are in conformity with national custom and tradition, rather than with any rule inherent within Tantrism itself.

In general, Indian scriptures recommend sun-enriched foods and urge yoga practitioners to avoid anything bitter, acid, strong-smelling or salty.

Typical counsel concerning food is that given in the Markandeya Purana:

"Rice gruel, buttermilk, barley, fruits, roots, saffron, porridge, oil cakes and raw grain flour—these foods are good for the yogi and lead to attainments. They should be eaten with concentrated mind and devoted care."

Like the ancient Greeks and Egyptians, Tantriks believe that during the more spiritually advanced ages which preceded the present one, men subsisted wholly upon fruits, grain and vegetables.

But they recognize that in this, the debased age of Kali, one's diet must sometimes include so-called tamasic foods, strictly eschewed by the spiritually advanced rishis who wrote the scriptures.

Too, the better-educated Shakta gurus take into account the fact that widely different diets are necessary to meet the requirements of various climates, customs, and ways of life.

"We take the view," explained Pundit Chatterjee, "that aside from a few solarized foods, good for anyone practicing Tantrik sadhana, you may eat whatever and whenever you wish. We are wholly in accord with the saying of Jesus that a man is not defiled by what goes into his mouth, but by what comes out of it.

"The chief consideration in the matter of eating," he

continued, "is to avoid anything that might seriously interfere with a fruitful practice of sadhana. It is only common sense to abstain from hard-to-digest foods when you are planning some activity that requires careful concentration and mental tranquility.

"In the West, the greater density of the spiritual magma (if I may use the term in that frame of reference), has led to overeating in attempts to cope with environment. Our practice of eating less at one time might be adopted with good results. My own guru taught that the stomach should be only one-fourth filled at breakfast, three-fourths at the noon meal; and one-half at the evening repast.

"On the other hand, I once met a sadhu who had attained extraordinary siddhi (supernormal powers), but whose belly was as big as that of Ganesha, from overeating.

"If you were to ask me to single out one food that, more than any other, is a Tantrik food, then I would say at once: honey. Mix it with ghee (clarified butter) in the proportion of three to one and take a tablespoonful morning and evening. Some years ago, the newspapers both here and abroad, carried an account concerning Srijut Malaviya, one of our prominent educators, who had discovered some secret of rejuvenation. It was reported that he had turned back the clock twenty years, so far as his personal appearance and vitality were concerned.

"I journeyed to Benares for the express purpose of learning from his own lips how he had accomplished it. When I pressed him for details, he told me that the chief dietary item in his remarkable discipline was honey mixed with ghee.

"An English student to whom I once imparted this information, wrote me after he had returned to England to say that he had found the same advice in his own scripture. It was written by the Hebrew rishi, Isaiah.[1]

"If we are to consider the subject of physical aids to sadhana in its broadest view, and from the standpoint of Western needs, there are other things equally as important as food.

Control of the body's polarity through exercise

"There is the matter of physical exercise, if I may mention one. In your country this usually means a more or less strenuous program, often at irregular intervals. The aim in view seems to be improved muscle tone, better circulation, and so on.

"For the follower of Tantra Shastra, the main purpose of exercise, as of all action, is greater control over the body's polarity. The spine is merudanda, that is to say, the static pole up and down which the dynamic currents of our earthly existence move. Therefore, we try by daily exercise to keep it flexible and vital.

"This is easily accomplished by walking at least one mile each day, always with the arms swaying, the palms facing forward. We also use familiar asanas such as halasan or yoga mudra, which you will find described in any popular book on Hatha Yoga.

1 Isaiah VII:15—"Butter and honey shall he eat, that he may know to refuse the evil, and choose the good."

"The Tantrik disciple is taught to give careful attention to his feet also—especially to the two large toes, for these are terminal points of important nadis. After bathing, they should be pulled, stretched and massaged with coconut oil, ghee or oil of almond, but never with anything containing animal fat.

"This procedure is perhaps even more important for you of the West than for Indian shisyas, because your feet are constantly encased in footwear of one kind or another. Here in India, as you have observed, we kick off our sandals at every opportunity. An American lady who visited our country recently said she is certain we are a nation of foot fetishists. Otherwise, how could one account for the fact that half our adult population are constantly massaging their bare feet or pulling their toes as they converse?

"Actually, I think they are acting from unconscious knowledge passed down to them by long-forgotten gurus of India's glorious past."

Pundit Chatterjee also had some suggestions for combating adverse effects of an urban, industrial environment. The polarity of our bodies, he said, is directly affected by our physical surroundings, and by the air we breathe.

The air of cities and industrialized areas is heavily charged with a positive polarity. Prolonged habitation in such an atmosphere produces the same physical effects as would result if the sadhaka permanently closed his left nostril and breathed only through the pingala or (right) sun channel. These effects include nervous tension, of which there is always a high incidence in big cities; vascular diseases, and emotional disorders.

One solution to this problem of urban living is for

the city dweller to increase the periods of breath flow through the ida or left nostril, as described earlier in the present work.

Another and obvious way is to take every opportunity to spend time in rural surroundings, especially in large open areas such as deserts, meadows, seashore or lake. Atmospheric ions, which are minute clumps of air molecules having an electrical charge, are negative in large open spaces of this kind. And being negative, they can often reverse the damage done by positive ions during sojourn in urban environment.

In this connection, it is interesting to observe that only recently, researchers both in the West and in Soviet Russia, have been seriously studying the effects of atmospheric polarity on human behaviour.

To date, their knowledge of this subject is not as extensive as that which has reposed in Tantrik tradition for centuries, but important experiments have been conducted under scientific test conditions.

At the Batelle Memorial Institute in Columbus, Ohio, where some of the tests were carried out, Drs. Howard G. Schultz and Richard A. Duffee pointed out that the effects of air ions on human health and behaviour have assumed a new importance in the nuclear, space age.

Observing that the astronaut and submariner may be exposed to ion concentrations considerably higher than normal, they said: "The effects of this increased ion concentration may be enhanced by other environmental factors such as stress."

Their experiments showed that negative ions produce a pleasant feeling of relaxation and drowsiness. Positively charged ions were found to produce an unpleasant feeling of dizziness and nausea, often accompanied by headache and sore throat.

The Russians also had space travel in mind when they launched a similar research project. The Soviet researchers reported that during the course of their study, athletes who inhaled negative ions during a period of fifteen minutes daily for twenty-five days, were able to grip a dynamometer 46% longer than control subjects not given the ions. After only nine days of negative ion treatment, treadmill endurance increased 55.9%.

If you are a city-dweller who cannot often get away to the wide-open spaces, you may, in a limited way, counteract the effects of your positively-charged atmosphere by walking barefoot through wet grass on your lawn, wading in pools or taking a plunge in a swimming pool or tub, provided the water is cool.

Water is negative and magnetic. Its effect, in perhaps a smaller measure, is the same as that of the sea or desert air—it relaxes tired nerves and eases tension.

On the other hand, walking barefoot upon the earth, especially through dust or sand, builds a positive polarity in your body.

In the matter of dress, Tantriks favor loose-fitting garments made of non-conductive material such as silk, wool, or linen. Most yogis regard tight-fitting Western clothes, especially those worn by men, with abhorrence.

In climates where the student is exposed to the hot sun's rays, he is cautioned to wear some kind of headgear which will protect the area at the base of his skull, where over-exposure to the sunlight can result in injury to his nervous system.

Tantra does not dwell at length upon the subject of physical fitness, as do some other systems of yoga. It is taken for granted that a *sadhaka* who seriously practices the disciplines given him by his guru will enjoy health —both mental and physical—regardless of his environment or social status.

Tantriks believe that, in the final analysis, health is nothing more than correctly balanced polarity. Such a balance brings harmony, first to the subtle body, then to the gross body and mind.

How is such harmony achieved?

There are several ways of changing polarity, some of which have already been presented. But to harmonize only during practice periods is not enough. A return to old ways of thinking and perspective following sadhana will mean a return to the same inharmony that created ill-health to start with.

The first requirement, then, is an over-all change of perspective. Such a change is not achieved by merely willing it. It comes, rather, through the realization that each of us has an individual purpose and destiny upon this earth.

Our daily lives are often filled with the trivial, the confused, the transient. But hidden within or beneath this seemingly meaningless activity is a pattern of light. This pattern of guided experience may be known only through intuitive awareness. Until such an awareness is achieved, the physical mind cannot think thoughts that soar to liberating heights above man's death world.

Illness, old age and death rule most men's inner thought. Their daily needs are measured to these. But a harmonious return to the soul's guided destiny releases to us a new outlook, because the poisonous fear of dissolution and misery is no longer the substance of our thought.

As a consequence, the physical body is liberated by relaxation of nerves and, through the *nadis,* is tuned to a higher vibration.

The soaring thought is a healing thought.

Therefore, hope and not fear, must be forever the ideal of living, if the *sadhaka* would conquer sickness and age—yes, even death.

> "All creation—gods, demons, universes—is the expansion of the Creator's thought into form. The nucleus of this is the substance of his mind. The power of projection is his will."
>
> —*Unpublished Text*

12. *The magic mirrors*

That portion of Tantrism presented in the foregoing chapters constitutes a methodology capable of universal application.

There is, however, another aspect of the system that for most Western students must remain strangely exotic and almost wholly within the realm of theory. That is the considerable part of Tantra which deals with *siddhi* or magical powers.

The main body of this secret knowledge is contained in such texts as the Indrajala Tantra or in the Damaras; in manuscripts buried deep within lamasary libraries in Tibet; and in oral traditions, transmitted only by word of mouth from guru to *shishya*.

Dangerous rituals and techniques

Most of the disciplines contain rituals and techniques far too dangerous to be presented in detail in a popular work such as the present one.

This does not preclude, however, the discussion, in a broad sense, of their nature and underlying principles.

Also, one or two typical disciplines that can be safely practiced by Western students, may serve to stimulate further interest and research.

The Christian and the Tantrik

There is, in fact, an urgent need for Western man to re-examine the whole concept of the supernatural in religious belief. A careful and honest evaluation of his faith may reveal to him that its mystical foundations are no longer tenable for him. At best, he will have to admit that he does not know where to draw the line between the credible and the incredible.

It is one of the illusions of the contemporary Western mind that Christianity will find a new lease on life if only its scriptures can be "demythologized."

Actually, such efforts at modernizing are, in the final analysis, merely admissions of pyrrhonism.

This growing and widespread disbelief is nowhere more evident than in the present-day skepticism among Christians concerning the miracles performed by Jesus and recounted in the New Testament.

How, for example, does the contemporary churchman explain the incident related in the Gospel of Matthew (XXI:19)?:

"And when he saw a fig tree in the way, he came to it and found nothing thereon, but leaves only, and said unto it, Let no fruit grow on thee henceforward forever. And presently the fig tree withered away."

Outside a Fundamentalist minority, most Christians either avoid stating an opinion, or, admitting that the Biblical record runs counter to scientific knowledge to-day, call for a new interpretation "to make the Gospel relevant to contemporary life."

The new interpretation does not, as did Tertullian, avail itself of the paradox. Tertullian declared:

"I believe because it is absurd . . . It is certain be-cause it is impossible."

However, it is not within the nature of the modern, Western personality to acknowledge anything as "real" which exists beyond the reach of reason, or outside the domain of physical law.

Accordingly, when confronted with stories of such irrational events as a crowd of five thousand being fed with five loaves and two fishes; or Lazarus raised from the dead, the educated Christian is obliged to adopt one of the following points of view:

1) The occurrence as described in the Biblical nar-rative did not really happen. The scriptural account is merely a legend, told to lend importance to the life and ministry of Jesus.

2) The "miracles" are really exaggerated accounts of natural happenings. E.g., Lazarus was not dead in the literal sense, but was mistaken for dead by his friends and relatives, while actually in a cataleptic state of suspended animation.

3) The stories of seemingly supernatural phenomena are really allegories used in exposition of spiritual truths. Hence, the story of Lazarus illustrates man's symbolical death, until he hears the voice of Jesus summoning him from the tomb of his sinful past. For did not Jesus himself elsewhere say, ". . . ye are like unto whited sepulchres, which indeed appear beautiful outward, but are within full of dead men's bones, and of all uncleanliness."

The Christian rationalist who believes that he has thus bridged the hiatus between Biblical record and scientific report, has in fact stopped short of the ultimate conclusions inherent in such a position.

For, carried to its logical extreme, rejection of the so-called miraculous element in religion becomes a rejection of religion itself, at least as religion is exemplified in the acts and utterances of Jesus of Nazareth.

What remains may be a noble way of life, but it is an ethic, not a revealed faith. Sooner or later, the Christian who is honest with himself will have to reject more than merely the wonderful deeds called miracles in his sacred texts.

To be consistent, he will also have to expel from his canon such familiar and fundamental practices as prayer. For is not prayer, in its commonly accepted sense, addressed to God, saints or intercessors—all supernatural entities?

Every supplication (including the oft-recited Lord's

Prayer) is magical in that it seeks to influence the "scientific" principles of cause and effect by asking divine intervention in human affairs.

On the secular, legal level, extirpation of the miraculous in our national life was achieved by the recent U.S. Supreme Court ruling that bans prayer in public schools.

Litigants, both individuals and groups, who successfully petitioned for this relief, were not motivated by fear of an established religion, or by desire for separation of church and state.

The secret and true dynamic of their action was the resolute determination to uproot from contemporary society the last vestiges of the supernatural.

The Tantrik and miracles

Viewed from a standpoint of calm detachment, the Western "believer" is thus a tragic and somewhat absurd figure, whose feverish involvement in social issues hides a poignant longing for a faith more spiritually fulfilling.

It is ironical that the non-Christian Tantrik would find no difficulty in accepting the miracle stories of the New Testament in their most literal sense.

One reason for this is the fact that he would not view them as miraculous in the same way that the Christian would. That is to say, the Tantrik would see them as natural events, produced by expert use of little-known forces. These forces, like everything in the universe, are but various manifestations of cosmic mind-stuff.

Shaktas believe that the ability to produce so-called psychic phenomena by means of this energy can be acquired by anyone who is willing to undergo the long and extremely arduous training necessary.

Jesus, in fact, made it clear that the "wonders" accomplished by him, could be duplicated by his disciples.

As the Tantrik conceives it, mind is the noumenal source of all phenomena. All aspects of creation, both visible and invisible are—regardless how tangible and objective they may seem to be in the physical world—only thought images projected by God or by other entities.

Psycho-mental energy

According to the secret lore, man can develop such concentration of mind that he is able to generate psycho-mental energy (called *rtsal* in Tibet) and to use it for bringing about results that to the unitiated appear to be supernatural.

It is because the Tantrik techniques employ these secret methods of concentration that Tantrism has been called the most elaborate system of auto-suggestion in the world.

While such an evaluation may serve to explain the more subjective visions of the *sadhaka*, it is hardly adequate to account for phenomena witnessed by persons other than the creator of them.

For example, Tantrik adepts (especially in Tibet) possess methods for projecting thought forms (called *tulpas*) which are materialized so completely that they are often mistaken for physical entities.

Moreover, these phantoms are sometimes vitalized and given a kind of autonomy, so that they may act and seemingly think without the consent or even the knowledge of their creator.

In this connexion, Madame Alexandra David-Neel, a Frenchwoman who spent many years among the lamas of Tibet, recounts an intriguing personal experience in creation of a *tulpa*.

Having a skeptical turn of mind, Madame David-Neel suspected that many stories she had heard concerning such materializations might be gross exaggerations.

The most common kind of *tulpa*-making in Tibet is that of forming and animating the counterparts of Tibetan deities. So, to avoid coming under the influence of this kind of mental suggestion—so prevalent around her—she chose for her thought child the figure of a fat, jolly monk.

After a few months of performing the prescribed disciplines for ritual projection of a thought image, Madame David-Neel relates that the form and character of her phantom monk took on the appearance of real life. He shared her apartment like a guest and when she departed for a journey, he accompanied her entourage.

At first, the monk put in an appearance only when his creator thought of him. But after a time, he began to behave in a very independent manner and to perform various actions not directed by his maker.

So real did he become in time, that on one occasion, when a herdsman came to the Frenchwoman's encampment to bring her some butter, he mistook the chimerical monk for a live lama.

Even more alarming to the phantom's begetter, his character began to undergo a subtle change. He grew leaner and his face gradually took on a sly, malevolent look. He daily grew more importunate and bold.

"In brief," says Madame David-Neel, "he escaped my control." [1]

Clearly, the time had come to purge herself of the unwanted companion whom she had brought to life, but who, by her own admission, had turned her existence into a day-nightmare.

It required six months of difficult practice and ritual to magically dissolve the monstrous prodigy.

"My mind-creature was tenacious of life," she declared.

How are we to explain such phenomena? Western psychology has only begun to investigate the secret and profound life of the mind. Many of their answers so far are far from adequate to account for occurrences such as that just cited.

The theory of hypnagogic hallucination is not satisfactory, since the image is clearly perceived by another person not aware of its existence.

Nor is the eidetic image explanation, which serves to clarify cases of children who have imaginary playmates that, for them, are real. Such invisible companions appear to be wholly subjective, although the annals of psychic research contain accounts of some in which adults have also seen the phantom playmate.

Be that as it may, in the case of the deliberately created phantom, such as Madame David-Neel's monk,

[1] David-Neel: "Magic and Mystery in Tibet."

the independence and individuality of the prodigy ought to give us considerable pause.

Even in the West, there have been instances in which thought images projected by one person, have been perceived and described by another who was totally unaware of the kind of mental picture projected.

An experiment of the kind was tried in France some time ago, with a satisfactory measure of success.

A person possessed of extraordinary powers of concentration was seated in a room opposite a plain white wall. He was asked to focus his attention upon the wall and to try to project upon it a certain mental image.

After a period of intense concentration, he left the room. A "sensitive"—that is, a person with highly developed faculty of extra-sensory perception—was then brought in.

The latter was instructed to concentrate upon the blank wall and to see whether he could detect the thought image projected upon it by his predecessor.

According to a published account of the experiment, the psychic clearly perceived and described phantom images upon the wall. It corresponded with that envisioned by the projector.

Tantrik texts assert that the universe all about us is teeming with thought forms and with beings good and bad—deities, demons, nature spirits, discarnate human egos, phantoms, monsters.

The *sadhaka* is not only made aware that they exist; he is taught disciplines that bring them under his control and enable him to communicate freely with them.

"Lady Cloud Walkers"

In Tibet, where rites aimed at this end (called *dubtobs*) still hold an important place in yogic practices, monks of several schools claim initiation by performance of the sex ritual with a female deity or Dakini. They aver that *maithuna* with a goddess of this kind results in bliss much more satisfying than that experienced when a mortal woman is the consort.

These Dakinis, who are also known as Khadomas or "lady cloud walkers," are the Tibetan equivalent of the Hindu *yakshis*. They are said to bestow great benefits upon the yogi who knows how and when to unite with them.

Indo-Tibetan texts devote considerable space to their praise and to descriptions of their beauty and grace of form. They are depicted as having finely-textured, ruby red skin; gentle, pensive faces; red eyes and finger nails; and are said to exude the faint fragrance of lotus blossoms.

On the walls of all Tantrik Tibetan temples will be found paintings (*thankas*) showing the Dakinis in both their benevolent and their wrathful aspects. In the latter form, they are sometimes portrayed as ferocious tiger-woman vampires, who feed on the flesh and blood of human victims. Others are naked, except for a ritual green scarf (*kata*) around their necks.

In a lower category of unearthly entities are nymph-like fairies, "white as lotus flowers, with pink eyes, and who are addicted to white, perfumed garments."

Tibetans believe these fairies sometimes incarnate as women. Consequently, they are much sought-after as ritual partners in lata-sadhana. The secret doctrine lists several special signs (physical characteristics) by which they may be identified.

"She-devils"

Other incarnating forces of Shakti take the forms of *lhamos* (she-devils), sorceresses, and *bhutas* (evil spirits).

It has been reported that some of the less enlightened "brothers of the hidden life" practice sex union with these she-devils; with discarnate human beings; and with phantoms whom they materialize for the purpose. Such practices are emphatically condemned by almost all gurus as being the lowest form of black magic.

Moreover, consorting with the latter class of entities is not without its dangers. Tantrik literature contains many warnings to the novice concerning the perils inherent in such intercourse. He is admonished that if these fiends escape his control, they may do him great harm, both physically and spiritually. Many Tibetan magicians construct thread-traps and magic cabinets to imprison them.

Four magical powers

And despite all warnings, Tibetans do not consider that a yogi has won his mystic spurs, so to speak, until he has pitted his thaumaturgic skill against that of various demons, and has acquired at least the classical *siddhis* or magical powers. These are:

1. *Shiwa*—the power to prevent misfortunes befalling oneself or others. It also includes the power of guarding against illness, and of prolonging the life-span.

2. *Gyaispa*—the so-called Expanding Yoga, by which power is attained to secure prosperity, fame, progeny and knowledge.

3. *Bangwa*—the Yoga of Ascendancy, by which the sadhaka controls assisting forces to influence man, animals, and inanimate objects. It also provides the means of attracting whatever one desires.

4. *Dragpo*—the Wrathful of Banishing Performance, the most terrible of all powers. By its disciplines, the yogi possesses the power to cause calamities, create enmity between human beings, kill and destroy; strike a person speechless, etc.

It is the *dragpo* techniques that are employed by the black magicians of Tibet who, unlike other Buddhists, believe in taking life and causing pain. Like their counterparts in the West—the Satanists—who employ an inverted crucifix and recite sacred liturgies backward, they intone the celebrated Tibetan mantra, "Om mani padme hum" in reverse.

Other *siddhi* or miraculous powers claimed by Tibetan mystics, as well as by a few Tantriks of India, include such things as: the ability to become invisible in a crowd; to walk upon water or through the air; to enter fire with immunity from burn; to walk long distances at incredible speed (called lung-gom); to know the thoughts of others; to yogically induce such great heat within the body that it will melt a snowfield; and to pass through walls or solid objects.

Two additional *siddhi* that are considered especially important in Tibet and deserve mention here, are those called *pho-wa* and *throng-jug.*

Briefly, pho-wa or the Yoga of Transference, is the mystic art of simulating the natural death process without fully and permanently cutting free from the body. That is to say, the yogi projects his consciousness or subtle body through the so-called Brahmananda (an aperture in the crown of the head), and travels about freely upon other planes of consciousness. It is a process similar to that known in the West as projection of the astral body.

An American neurologist, Dr. Andrija Puharich, who is conducting a remarkable program of scientific research in this and related fields, refers to the projected self as the "nuclear mobile center of consciousness." He relates the story of a prominent New York radio producer who experienced the pho-wa state when he accidentally inhaled some glue he was using in the construction of a cabinet in his children's room.[1]

In the case of Pho-wa, however, the out-of-body consciousness is not left to wander indiscriminately, but is strictly disciplined and set to accomplishing definite objectives.

One of the latter is to assist dying persons with a kind of spiritual guidance that directs their entrance into the Bardo plane—the state intermediate between death and rebirth. Details of this discipline have been discussed at length in several books available to the general public. The most authoritative and complete of these is "The Tibetan Book of the Dead," an English translation of

[1] Andrija Puharich, M.D.: "Beyond Telepathy."

which has been arranged and edited by the well-known Oxford scholar, W. Y. Evans-Wentz.

Thron-jug involves some of the same procedure as that of Pho-wa, but is more difficult and requires greater advancement on the part of the yogi who performs it.

Essentially, *thron-jug* is the projection of one's consciousness into, and the taking over of, another human body. Adepts who claim that power, assert that by means of it they can temporarily discard their own body and take over the body of another person—either one who has just died, one asleep, or even a casual passerby.

There are many stories told in both India and Tibet of various feats of *thron-jug*, performed by great initiates of the past, such as Shankara in India and Marpa in Tibet. Just how factual these accounts are must be a matter left to the individual judgment of each person who hears them.

As for the practice of pho-wa and thron-jug, all gurus are in agreement upon one point: it is a highly dangerous operation. By repeatedly projecting oneself outside the body, they warn, the yogi gradually loosens the bonds holding him to his fleshly abode. These may eventually be dissolved altogether and the performer find himself without a physical body.

There are other hazards, too. While one is absent from his body, the subtle link still connecting the nuclear self to the physical form, may be broken, in which case ordinary death occurs.

Also, there is the outside chance that powerful discarnate entities, human or demoniac, may forcibly enter and possess the vacated body. In many cases of insanity, according to the Tibetan theory, such possession has occurred.

For these, and other reasons, Tantrik gurus include the secret art of pho-wa and thron-jug among those teachings called tam-gyud, which constitute the "whispered tradition,"—instruction that is always transmitted orally from teacher to disciple.

Although a number of Tantrik teachings are thus considered too dangerous to be committed to the written or printed word, others have been preserved in manuscript form. These manuscripts and Tibetan block prints have been copied many times, often with annotations or commentary added.

To give the reader some idea of the power and purpose of practices contained in this secret lore, the following exercise will be useful. It is performed for the purpose of materializing in the physical plane, anything strongly desired.

FIFTH DISCIPLINE

The sadhana may be practiced at any time, day or night. However, most gurus say it is more effective when performed before sunrise, in the early morning hours.

Either Eastern or Western posture may be used, so long as the spine is kept arrow-straight. The yogi faces the East. If the cross-legged *asana* of India is assumed, the sadhaka ought to sit on a folded blanket or some kind of padding.

To prepare for the dynamic part of the exercise, he breathes in and out rhythmically to the 7:1:7:1 count employed in early disciplines.

After completing twelve cycles of this ratio (or more,

if needed to clear the passages), the postulant relaxes for a moment and allows the breath to flow as it will.

He then grasps the left wrist and upper portion of the back of the left hand with his right hand. With the hands joined in this way, he places them palms downward over the Navel Chakra or transformation center, at the solar plexus.

As explained elsewhere, Tantriks attach great importance to this chakra. It is regarded as a kind of psychic power plant, in which is generated the mystic fire that Tibetans call *tumo*.

The sadhaka now closes his eyes and visualizes within this center a tiny, intensely brilliant tongue of flame. It should be imagined as being no larger than a hair-thin, incandescent wire, twisted at the top like a corkscrew.

When this image has become clearly established in the mind's eye, the yogi begins once more to breathe slowly and deeply, using again the 7:1:7:1 rhythm.

As the breath flows in and out, he thinks of his lungs as a bellows, stoking the glowing tongue of fire within the Navel Chakra until it incandesces more and more.

After a time, a soft warmth will envelop the region of the solar plexus. At that point, the yogi substitutes for his image of the *tumo* fire, a mental picture of the thing or condition desired by him.

Then, by breathing in and out in short, staccato spurts, he causes his abdomen and diaphragm to move back and forth in quick, spasmodic motion, as one does when sobbing. Meanwhile, the desired visualization is continued.

This portion of the exercise lasts for perhaps two minutes during which the sadhaka concentrates intensely upon the desired objective. Then he lowers his head until his chin presses firmly against his chest. All the air is expelled from the lungs, and the breath is held outside for a count of seven. His hands (still clasped in the mudra described above) press the solar plexus and shake that area with a quick, vibrating motion, such as would be produced by an electric reducing belt.

While doing this, he again strongly visualizes his desire, bringing it into sharp focus within his mind.

"Having thus awakened the spirit essence of his desire within himself," says one text, "the yogi once again inhales. As he does so, he raises his head upward, until he is gazing at the ceiling or sky."

Then, tensing the muscles of his throat to lock the breath (prana) within, he forces the air quickly downward until it presses hard against the diaphragm and the navel chakra.

Holding the breath for a count of seven, the yogi visualizes the *tumo* flame entering the central canal of his spine (the *shushumna*) and passing upward toward the crown of the head. With it, he sends the mental substance of his desire.

As he exhales, he imagines his desire to be outside himself. It has now become an exteriorized, living thought form, objective and real.

The first time the discipline is practiced, the sadhaka usually does not repeat it more than three times. But on successive occasions, as he strengthens his desire-image, he may perform as many as seven cycles.

He persists in the practice until the desired objective is fully realized, even if the effort requires many months or years. One of the chief virtues of the Tantrik is perseverance, and constancy in the performance of any given discipline.

"One of the chief obstacles in the path of Western students," said Pundit Chatterjee, "is their impatience. They are so accustomed to a push-button society in which effect follows cause with lightning speed, they expect instant results from their sadhana.

"But in the Shiva science we have to do with another order of existence—that of the inner planes, where time as we know it does not exist. An event may happen instantaneously, in a year, or in a *kalpa*. Or simultaneously in all these.

"Therefore, *sadhana*—if performed rightly and persistently—will surely bear fruit in its proper season and according to divine plan, not man's.

"If I say to an Indian *shishya*, 'Repeat this mantram a crore (100,000) of times,' he sets himself to the task without complaint. But if I tell a Western student that to be successful in an undertaking, he must recite a single syllable a thousand times, he looks upon it as a great burden."

A Tibetan lama recently made an observation similar to that of Pundit Chatterjee concerning the time lapse which often ensues between the setting in motion of psychic forces and visible results.

He had been asked by a Western newsman why, if Tibetan naljorpas (wizards) possess the supernatural powers they claim, they permitted the Chinese Communists to occupy their country and to drive the Dalai Lama into exile.

"The chronicle is not yet closed," he replied. "We have released an invisible army of the *dharmapalas* (guardian demons) against our foe. Terrible suffering and defeat will yet come to the invader—those who pollute the pure Land of Snows (Tibet), and those who support the godless government in Peking."

Even as the yogi is acquiring and using the forces of creation, however, he is called upon to meditate constantly upon the unreality of their nature.

The Buddhist tradition, especially, reminds him that he as he appears in this world, and all he creates here, are aggregates of individual elements and, as such, doomed to dissolution in time.

There is nothing that he can hold forever as his own, nothing he can create that will not change and vanish. Dream and dreamer are devoid of enduring substance and true entity. His occult powers (siddhi) are but magic mirrors in which are reflected fleeting images—as the moon in water, a cloud in the sky, a rainbow across heaven—vivid and beautiful, but having no self-substance.

For the end of all this is the Great Silence, the unfathomable womb of Shakti.

> "The night-time of the body is the daytime of the
> Soul."
>
> —*Tantrik Saying*

13. *Yoga of the dream state*

Each of us, according to Tantrik traditions, lives not
one, but two lives, simultaneously.

One is the objective, physical life of the five senses.
It is our waking life, lived here and now, limited by time
and space. It is the life you return to each morning
when you open your eyes, and the familiar "solid" objects of your room—lamps, table, chairs—recall to you
the frustrations, restraints, and insecurities of the world
that dissolved in sleep.

Our "second life"

The second life is that which is lived "over there," in the so-called dream world which we enter when we fall asleep. It is an existence very different from that we lead in our workaday sphere.

For, as Indo-Tibetan scriptures point out, the rational existence we know when awake does not exist there. It is, rather, a world of free exaltation. We take to the air like birds, walk through walls, change physical form as easily as smoke. We are like children at play—full of whimsy, sly mischief, and fairy-like delights.

In the Brihadaranyaka Upanishad, it is written:

"Having subdued by sleep all that belongs to the body, he not asleep himself, looks down upon the sleeping senses. Having taken to himself light, he goes again to his place—the golden person, the lonely swan.

"Guarding his lower nest with the vital breath, the immortal moves away from the nest. The immortal one goes wherever he likes, the golden person, the lonely bird.

"Going up and down in the dream state, the god makes many forms for himself, enjoying himself in the company of women, or laughing (with his companions), or beholding terrible sights . . .

"Here some people (object and) say:

" 'This state of sleep is the same as his waking state, for whatever objects he sees while awake, those too, he sees when asleep.'

"Not so, for in the dream state, the person is self-illuminated."

It is interesting to observe that even at the early date (circa 1000 B.C.) at which this scripture was written, the sages anticipated a point of view that is commonly held today. That is the theory that the content of all our dreams is derived from impressions, incidents, and mental experiences of our waking life.

Not so, say the sacred texts. The golden person, that is, the individual self, leaves the body (called "the lower nest") and, clothed in spiritual integument as mobile and penetrating as radio waves, exists in another dimension.

This dimension differs in many strange ways from that in which our earthly lives are unfolded. Tibetan mystics say that it closely resembles the intermediate *Bardo* state of the discarnate ego, between death and rebirth. For that reason they refer to it as Bardo of the Dream.

They assert that the ego's shock of re-entry, so to speak, which occurs when we return to the dense physical realm upon awakening from sleep, usually shatters and distorts accurate memory of dream experiences.

This fact, added to the wholly different conditions of life in that other sphere, make our dreams, in retrospect, seem unreal, illogical and sometimes downright silly.

One factor that contributes a great deal to the confusion of dreams is that of so-called time distortion. Time as we know it in our waking experiences, is conceived as an irreversible direction, a sequence of moments at which given events occur.

But on the inner planes, adepts report that the distinction between past, present and future does not exist. Time is simultaneous; and the vivid present as we experience it in physical realms, is at best a point of arbitrary awareness by the dreamer.

If the dreamer so desires, or if he permits astral world

nature to take its course, he may view the total history of anything having measurable duration.

For example, he may see a person, or his own physical counterpart, in every stage of temporal development, from infancy to old age.

This circumstance may, to some extent, answer the question that so often puzzles the plain man when he tries to visualize life after death, either in a Christian framework of reference positing a timeless hereafter; or in the metaphysical sense, seeking to formulate some image of a disembodied ego. Each asks, What age will I be over there? A child, a youth, a middle-aged person, a Methuselah?

Any and all of these, say those who have learned how to bring back lucid interpretations of that different order of existence which obtains in other worlds than ours.

It is true that, being to some extent in control of the time flow during the dream state, most of us prefer youth, as we do in our waking state. Mark Twain, who was firmly convinced that his spiritualized body wandered the universe during the interval of sleep, wrote that he was always young in his dreams.

Another faculty denied us in the third dimension, but fully exercised in the dream state, is the ability to see through "solid" objects. Such capability is not confined to the imponderable things of the subtle planes, but apparently can function even in the gross world.

X-ray vision of this kind is well illustrated in the case, often cited amongst occultists, of the French naturalist, Jean Louis Agassiz.

Agassiz had, for two weeks, been puzzling over the faint impression of a fossil fish in a slab of stone. But, try as he might, he could not make out distinct outlines of the primordial creature's structure. Unable to classify the specimen, he put the project aside and busied himself with other problems.

Soon afterward, however, he awakened in the small hours with the impression that during his sleep, he had again examined the stone fragment, only, this time he had clearly seen complete details of the fish's configuration. What had it looked like? He pressed his memory for particulars. But to no avail. Only a blurred image remained.

Hoping to stimulate even this vague recollection and perhaps to recapture some of the missing features presented in his dream experience, Agassiz again studied the specimen with utmost concentration. But it was hopeless. He could remember nothing.

The following night, he again saw the fish in his dreams. But again, the "trauma" of awakening erased the details.

Determined to set down the vision if possible, the moment it occurred, Agassiz thoughtfully provided himself with a pencil and paper on his bedside table.

In the early hours of the following morning, the dream did recur. He seemed to be peering intently at the fossil specimen. At first, only the blurred outlines, observed during his waking research, were visible to him. But gradually his gaze penetrated the stone until he could plainly see the fundamental characteristics of the ancient fish, embedded deep within the stone, beyond waking vision.

Half awake, he groped in the darkness for the paper and pencil at his bedside. Finding these, and without putting on a light, he sketched the skeletal profile of the specimen as he had just witnessed it in his dream.

His wife relates that when he awakened the following morning, he was surprised, upon examining the drawing, to discover hidden features of the fish, which he had not expected to find. They had been concealed inside the stone itself.

Realizing that only a kind of x-ray vision could have revealed these to him, M. Agassiz hurried to the Jardin des Plantes to verify his discovery.

Using his dream sketch as a guide, he patiently chiseled away a section of the stone. And there, concealed beneath its surface, was the portion of the organism hitherto invisible to him. It corresponded in every detail with the drawing he had made in the almost total darkness of his bedroom the previous night!

Yoga of the dream state

Thus, while ordinarily our memory of dreams is a rambling, irrational and meaningless confusion, it must be evident to the unbiased reader that in some instances, as in the case of M. Agassiz, the dream experience can and does have important meaning for the dreamer.

Such a theory provides the basis for yoga of the dream state, as we shall see in what follows.

Sometimes the dream experience is so real and overwhelming (especially in the case of vaticinal dreams) that it will overshadow our thoughts for hours or days after we emerge from sleep.

A well-known instance of such a premonitory dream

is that which occurred to Abraham Lincoln a few days before he was assassinated. A vivid account of it is given in the biography, "Recollections of Abraham Lincoln," written by Ward Hill Lamon, one of the President's most intimate friends.

In his dream, President Lincoln told Lamon, he heard the subdued sobbing of many people, seemingly in deep grief. He arose from his bed and wandered from room to room, seeking the source of the weeping. He said every room was illuminated, and he could clearly see the familiar furnishings. But, though the sound of mourning filled the house, he did not meet a single person as he passed along.

With growing bafflement and a feeling of alarm, the President continued his search through the White House until he entered the East Room. There he was shocked to see a corpse resting upon a catafalque. It was guarded by soldiers and surrounded by a crowd of mourners. The face of the deceased was covered, and the President asked one of the soldiers:

"Who is dead in the White House?"

"The President," he replied. "He was killed by an assassin."

At this point, a loud outburst of weeping by the crowd awoke Mr. Lincoln. But the dream, so soon to come true, haunted his remaining days on earth.

It was not the first time, of course that a great man of destiny or genius has had a premonitory vision in his sleep. There is, running through the recorded history of every culture, a long list of prophetic dreams, beginning with the famous fat-and-lean kine dream of the Pharaoh of Egypt, accurately interpreted for him by Joseph.

Other celebrated Biblical narratives of prophetic dreams include those of Jacob and his ladder; Nebuchadnezzar and the dream he couldn't remember, although God revealed it to Daniel "in a night vision"; and Joseph, the husband of Mary, who was warned in a dream to take the infant Jesus and flee into Egypt.

For the reader interested in a comprehensive history of the subliminal life, there is a vast body of literature, ancient and modern, dealing with the subject in almost all its aspects.

Some accounts tell of the important role played by dreams in the creative life of writers, composers, scientists, and even financiers.

Others relate documented instances in which the dreamers were given cures for illness, locations of buried treasure or lost objects, diagnosis of an unsuspected pathology, solution of a mathematical problem, telepathic messages, and so on.

For the ancients, however, the primary importance of the dream process was that it provided a doorway into the spiritual realm, a means of communication between man and higher assisting forces. The Hebrew believed that God himself could speak to man in a dream.

"In a dream, in a vision of the night," wrote Job (33:15–18), "when deep sleep falleth upon men, in slumberings upon the bed; then he openeth the ears of men, and sealeth their instruction, that he may withdraw man from his purpose, and hide pride from man, he keepeth back his soul from the pit, and his life from perishing by the sword."

Similarly, the true objective of dream yoga, as practiced by Tantrik sadhakas is to preserve a continuity of awareness in the dream state, and thereby to reach beyond the confusions and elusive images of ordinary sleep.

For the Tantrik sleep is, in fact, a form of samadhi, closely resembling that claimed by yogis who practice extreme austerities to achieve it.

Tantrik gurus point out that it is no coincidence that in inducing the classical state of samadhi, the yogi more or less duplicates the mechanism of sleep. He slows the rhythm of his breath, regulates and deepens his respiration. He effects a general relaxation of the muscles. By inhibiting the nerve centers, the threshold of awareness that responds to stimuli is raised, as it is in sleep. Moreover, the electrical activity of the brain during samadhi, as measured by the electroencephalograph, shows the same characteristics as those recorded during deep sleep.

In short, if ordinary sleep can provide a ready means of reaching higher planes of consciousness (provided the proper method is applied), the non-ascetic Tantrik believes such a technique is the proper one for men of the Kali age.

Obstacles to the successful practice of dream yoga are somewhat the same as those which confront the Western investigators of "the buried life."

The first problem is how to separate dreams having their origin in sensuous impressions and experiences of waking life, from those of spiritual significance.

Long before modern researchers in Europe and America began an extensive study of dreams, Indo-Tibetan schools were aware that dreams can be caused by such things as over-eating or improper diet; by stimulation of any of the sleeper's five senses; wish fulfillment, and so on.

Scientifically trained investigators in the West, who have propounded their various dream theories with the fervor of fanatics, condescendingly regard yogic dream practices as mystic nonsense, when they know anything about them at all. They assume that Tantrik teachers hold the views they do because of their ignorance of Occidental experimentation and study.

So far as the better-educated gurus are concerned, nothing could be further from the truth.

Pundit Chatterjee, for example, was fully conversant with the work of such modern authors as Freud, Jung, Janet, Adler, Brill and Lowy. He could also speak knowledgeably of studies being conducted by medical researchers, among them Hess, Mazurkiewitz, Loomis, and the Gibbses.

Three states of consciousness

"We who receive our light from the Sadhana Shastra do not reject the data of science," he said. "But we say they stop short of the subtle and secret matters that concern us.

"It may well be that some dreams are confessions, as Stekel claims. And we know that dreams can be produced experimentally or affected by tensor effects, orientation to surroundings, antecedent states of mind, pathology, perhaps even genetic memory from the far-distant past.

"Again: they speak truthfully when they say that dreams are often ridiculous, disconnected, trivial, repetitious, improper, and sometimes even criminal. But we believe they are wrong to affirm that they are always so.

"Our revealed literature declares that there are three states of consciousness for the embodied Jiva. One is the state of being in this world of forms; one in the other, formless world; and the third, in an intermediate realm —*sandhyam,* in which we experience at the same time the evils of the gross world and the joys of the subtle world. It is this intermediate state of consciousness that produces the irrational, grotesque and incongruous dreams of which science has made so careful a study.

"In the sacred text, we find it written: 'When this person goes to sleep, he carries with him the material of this all-embracing world. In the dream condition, he tears it apart, himself builds it up. He sleeps (that is, dreams) by his own light. In that state, the person becomes self-illuminated. He is, indeed, the creator (of his dreams).'

"Is this all that is to be said of the dream state? Certainly not. Tantrik Acharyas have long taught that by the right discipline, the yogi passes beyond the irrational, intermediate state, into clear awareness of the other world."

Dream yoga has two principal aims. One is initiatory; the other liberating.

The secret order of epoptae

The cryptic scriptures of Tantrism speak of a secret, universal order of epoptae, who can initiate a sleeping aspirant anywhere in the world.

It is said that the powerful lines of force emanating from their transcendental consciousness may be perceived at any point in the universe. In the postulant, they produce certain dream experiences, which he must remember, analyze, and absorb.

Some of these adepts embody the Shiva or male *purusha* principle; while others incarnate one or another of the many aspects of the Devi—the dynamic, creative female force called *prakriti*.

Disciplines employed in these initiations are reportedly the same as those imparted to the disciple when the guru is present in the physical body. They include purification, breath control (pranayama), mantra, *nyasa* or projection of divine entities into various parts of the body; *dhyana* (yogic meditation); and *panchatattva* (the secret ritual). The sexual partner for the latter practice may be the guru projecting in the guise of almost any personality, East or West; past, present, or future.

Or, according to Tibetan sources, Tantrik deities such as Dakinis or Devas may serve as consorts.

Whether these claims be true or not, all teachers of dream yoga start their instruction with techniques for remembering dreams and for analyzing dream symbols. The *shishya* is trained to use his waking consciousness as a cognitive mechanism, endlessly scanning for truth recorded in the memory of dreams.

In thus seeking in dreams for a source of instruction and guidance, the Tantrik tradition is not an isolated discipline. Study and interpretation of this kind has a long antecedent history.

The ancient Chaldean sages, the "Wise Men of the Magic Library" in Egypt; the Magi of Persia; the dream oracles of Greece—all held important positions in their respective societies because they had developed the techniques of comprehnding dreams and of delivering messages of divine origin when they concerned the people as a whole.

The Roman Caesar Augustus believed firmly in mantic dreams, and had a law enacted which required the citizens of certain provinces to publish in the marketplace any dream they might have concerning the State.

In the Islamic world, Mohammed, who was a reformer in some matters—social and religious—reaffirmed the dream process as part of the prophetic mission.

It is said that each morning he used to ask his followers to relate to him their dreams of the previous night and to analyze them for anything that might be of a revelatory nature. Tibetan gurus follow the same procedure today on occasions when a disciple is to receive initiation.

In the Indo-Tibetan tradition, various formulas have been developed for the purpose of removing the "defilements" that veil the true dream content, beclouding one's awareness during initiations that occur in sleep.

The following technique, devised for Western disciples by Pundit Chatterjee, is based upon classical traditions:

SIXTH DISCIPLINE

The first step in the discipline of dream yoga is preparatory. That is to say, the sadhaka seeks to create the optimum conditions conducive to his comprehending and remembering dream experiences.

He should, therefore, first be mindful of his own physical and mental state. If he leads a sedentary life, he ought to take a short, brisk walk in the fresh air before retiring, in order to relax his muscles. On the other hand, strenuous exercise that results in fatigue, is to be avoided.

The final meal of the day ought to be a light one, free of rich or stimulating dishes. If coffee or tea interfere with sleep, they ought to be eschewed.

A pleasant state of mind, free of daily cares and worldly anxieties, is a sine qua non in the practice of dream yoga. Therefore, the sadhaka must achieve tranquillity, either by pranayama, by reading, or by listening to the kind of music he has individually found to be relaxing and calming to his nerves.

He should also direct his attention to the room in which he is to sleep. It should be of pleasing, but subdued décor. The colors most desirable for his purpose are pastel shades of blue or green. Bright primary colors —red, yellow, blue—are the most inappropriate for a room in which to practice.

It should also be a quiet room, insulated against traffic sounds and noises that are likely to prove intrusive during hours of slumber. The auditory, more than the other physical senses, is susceptible to stimulation during sleep, owing to the fact that there is a rise and fall in its acuteness, as the sadhaka's sleep lightens or deepens at intervals during the night.

The room should be well-ventilated, but not flooded with cold night air. The sleeper would likewise be protected against excessive light which, in controlled experiments, has been found to produce retinal images and phantasies that, of course, interfere with the yogi's aim of contacting higher consciousness.

After a careful check of himself and of the room in which he will sleep, the aspirant examines his bed. The mattress should be neither too hard nor too soft; that is to say, it should be of a resiliency that will not affect the dreamer's subliminal consciousness.

Squeaky springs or a bedstead that creaks and groans with the slightest movement of the sleeper's body likewise constitutes a serious drawback to practice. A sound barely noticed in the waking state sometimes brings on alertness in a person who happens to be in a light state of sleep at the time.

An average person will move an arm or a leg perhaps twenty or thirty times during an eight-hour period of rest; and make as many as fifteen complete body turns during that same period. If his bed-springs twang, or his headboard gives forth a strident protest at each movement, the sadhaka is not likely to realize a successful sadhana.

Selection of a pillow is also important. It ought to be of a thickness that will support the head at an angle to the body that will not produce neck strain. A thin notebook, used for the present purpose only, and a pencil are placed beneath the pillow, where they can be easily found in the darkness.

The bed linens should be fresh and clean, and free of wrinkles and bulges. The pillow case may be scented with the sadhaka's favorite fragrance, or any of the perfumes noted in Chapter 7.

If blankets are tucked under the mattress at the foot of the bed, they must be loose enough so as not to be binding to the sleeper's lower limbs.

Finally, the feet must be kept warm, even if it is necessary to wear woolen bed socks during the colder months in northern climates.

After the foregoing details have been attended to, the yogi proceeds to the second step of the discipline.

Getting into bed, and with lights extinguished, he lies at first on his back, eyes closed and hands folded over the solar plexus, as directed in the Fifth Discipline.

For a few moments, he lies quite still, breathing normally and relaxing as fully as possible, both mentally and physically. If he is accustomed to saying a prayer upon retiring, he does so now.

Then, arousing an intense desire to attract higher assisting forces from the inner planes, he resolves to retain a continuity of awareness through the dream state. This awareness will clearly enable him to recall his dreams in the waking state.

A drowsiness begins to overcome the sadhaka. He assumes the supine posture, called by Tibetan Tantriks the Lion Posture, as follows: Lying on his right side, with his head to the North, he pulls up his legs slightly until both knees are bent. In this position, the left leg lies atop the right one. He places his right cheek in the cupped palm of his right hand, and rests his left arm along the left leg.

If, during the ensuing period of sleep, he unconsciously moves out of this position, it need give him no serious concern. The important thing is to fall asleep in that posture.

Immediately upon awaking, whether it be the following morning or at different times during the night, the sadhaka records details of his dream or dreams in the notebook placed under his pillow for that purpose.

Even though only vague fragments of the dream are still present, these should be noted. The notes are made before fully opening the eyes, while still in the limbo between the *svapna* (sleeping) and the *jagrat* (waking) states.

If only a few disconnected features of the dream are available, he ought to try to start with the seemingly latest image and work backward, trying to fully relive the dream experience a second time. The complete dream scenario may, in this way, pass again through the yogi's memory.

The image or incidents that come most sharply into focus are duly described in the notebook. This done, an earnest effort is made to recall his own participation in the dream: what he did, said, heard.

Careful attention is given to anything extraordinary about the dream content—images or identities or places which, although they seemed perfectly natural in the subliminal milieu, appear startling or impossible in the waking state.

Until he has recovered as much as possible of the total dream sequence, the sadhaka does not allow himself to return fully to wakefulness or to think of anything other than the dream he is trying to recall.

Having recaptured and revisualized his dream as fully as possible, he records the date and puts the notebook aside.

In the event that upon awaking, the sleeper is unable to recall any part of his dream, he should try to recall what his first conscious thought was, upon emerging from sleep. This thought, no matter how trivial and seemingly irrelevant, is very often closely associated with the just-concluded dream experience. It can therefore serve as a connecting link, which will bring back other details.

Tantrik teachers say that difficulty in remembering dreams may come from too sudden an awakening. They urge their disciples to check for conditions that may cause precipitous or premature awakening. These include such things as bodily tension, extremes in temperature, noise, chronic alertness.

To overcome the latter obstacle, the sadhaka is told to visualize a brilliant blue, almond-shaped flame glowing in the *muladhara* or sex chakra. As he meditates upon it, he pictures the electric-blue fire radiating outward along the 72,000 *nadis* or psychic channels of his subtle body, until it envelops his gross body in a luminous cloud.

It is not unusual for the normal person to awaken one or more times during the night. The reason for this is that our sleep is not an unbroken period of unconsciousness. It is, rather, made up of six or seven sleep intervals, separated by shallow slumber or outright wakefulness. Each sleep cycle lasts slightly more than an hour, in the same way that the breath flow alternates from *ida* to *pingala*.

If the yogi does come fully awake during the night, he tries each time to recall his dream and to record it in his notebook.

Most Tantrik gurus hold the view that dreams which are important from a yogic point of view, are more likely to occur between dawn and sunrise. It is not difficult to see why. At that time the physical body has had its rest, all food has been digested, and the mind has been largely cleared of "defilements," that is, of residual sense impressions.

After faithfully recording his dreams for a week or ten days, the postulant goes over them carefully, studying each image or impression. Of particular interest are scenes that appear to be out of another age, or in surroundings that bear little resemblance to those of the dreamer's waking life. Close attention is given to the sifting of data that include meetings, conversations, or unusual mutual activities with persons or beings unknown to the sadhaka in the physical world.

Especially noteworthy are dream experiences of a sexual nature. These may not at first be recognized for what they are. They may appear initially in symbol. In the latter form, however, they will always involve imagery representing a union of opposites, such as electric and magnetic, hot and cold, light and dark, static and kinetic. For example, the dream may be of a merry-go-round, in which a static pole supports the movement, and makes possible a variety of activity around it.

The student must bear in mind, of course, that these dreams have more than one level of significance. They may, indeed, be the expressions of unfulfilled desires, as Freud asserts; or arise from the collective unconscious, as Jung avows.

But deeper than these sources, for the Tantrik, lies another genesis of his dream: his need to reintegrate the opposite poles of his being, into a Nirvanic unity.

Eventually, if sleep sadhana is successful, the symbolization process will give way to a direct relationship with another person or being, usually of the opposite sex.

"The *saha-dharmini* (ritual consort) may appear to the dreamer in many guises," Pundit Chatterjee observed. "For the Hindu man or woman, it may be as

Parvati, Kali, Durga, Shiva or Vishnu. For the Tibetan, the embodiment may be of the Dakinis or the Yidam. For you of the West, it is less likely to be a goddess or religious figure. For you, the form taken may be a casual stranger, a movie star, the girl next door.

"Shastra teaches that Shiva-Shakti may take any form, being the fountainhead of all forms. Therefore, the sadhaka ought to meditate upon this before falling asleep. He ought to repeat again and again: 'O my Shakti, come to me, come to me, come to me!' He should also try to visualise each stage of the Secret Act with that one who has clearly manifested to him in the *svapna* (dream) state."

According to Tantrik belief, if the neophyte persists in his practice, sooner or later an initiator will emerge from the shifting and amorphous experiences of his dreams.

Until he has clearly identified such an initiator, he is required to continue the dream record in his note-book, and to scan it carefully for important data he may have overlooked.

When the initiator or unifying element of the dream state has been discovered, the yogi is ready for the next step of the present discipline.

This consists of what is called the Practice of the Return. Each time the initiating element—whether it be person, symbol, color, sound—is remembered upon awakening, the aspirant with eyes still closed continues to visualize the key image and to return to the dream.

In other words, he seeks to repeat the entire dream, but to carry into it his waking consciousness, with the latter's lucidity and self-control.

He thus becomes a detached spectator, as well as a

participant in the unfolding experience. He will reason about the strange scenes before him as one might reason about a motion picture drama evolving upon a screen before him.

He may at first find this difficult to accomplish, since it means being in two worlds simultaneously. But after patient and repeated attempts, a successful transfer of mundane consciousness to the inner planes will occur.

Then, Tantrik adepts assert, the dreamer—freed of all trammels of the flesh, although still umbilical to the body by means of a nuclear ribbon—will emerge from his old, familiar surroundings and enter a universe ruled by different laws (*kaivalya*).

Then and there, his preceptor and guide will take over to conduct him through the rites of *diksha*.

Dream-state disciplines of Tibetan Buddhist Tantriks differ in some respects from those of India. The lamas teach that all sensorial impressions of both waking and dream states are equally illusory. The only distinction between the two states is that one is external, the other subjective. But, as the Hindu scripture has said, the whole world is the dream of Brahma. When Brahma wakes, the dream ends.

Only by learning to pierce this veil of unreality, by comprehending his dreams, can the sadhaka awaken to the True State of Enlightenment.

Consequently, the aim of Tibetan sleep sadhana is to prepare the disciple to recognize clearly and to hold the Four Blisses which emerge both in the dream experience and in the after-death state.

These four successive unfoldments are known as the Lights of Sleep. The first, called the Light of Revelation, is perceived either just before or during the early stages of sleep. It resembles effulgent, moth-white moon-light in a cloudless sky.

As the feeling of drowsiness deepens, the admixture of residual sense impressions and discriminating thoughts begins to subside. At that point the second illumination, known as the Light of Augmentation, dawns. It appears to the Jiva usually as brilliant clear sunlight. During the dying process, it marks the stage referred to as the time of Ignition.

Only advanced yogis are able to proceed beyond this stage, to comprehend the two remaining Lights. For those who can, however, the sunlight fades into total darkness, like an eclipse. This is the Light of Immediate Attainment. As the sleeping sadhaka learns to meditate upon it, he will perceive a dim glow, "like the light of a lamp enclosed in a semi-opaque vessel."

The Light of Immediate Attainment dissolves as the yogi plunges deeper into profound slumber. It merges into the ultimate Void, or Innate Light, described as the primal radiance of all Reality. From it comes the light and heat of the sun, and the reflected brilliance of the moon.

"Here in the fourth degree of Voidness, abides the Son of Mother Clear Light," declares a Tibetan treatise, "until he rises out of it, as a fish leaping forth from water, and passes forthwith into enlightenment."

It must be evident to the reader that the Tibetan discipline is, in fact, a rehearsal for the final sleep called death. Lamaic scriptures teach that the Bardo of Death, which comes at the end of every human life is identical with the Bardo of the Dream. Having died nightly many times, the sadhaka who has learned the yogic art of

Emergence, passes into the after-death state with the same ease with which he enters the dream world.

Sir Thomas Browne, in his "Religio Medici," expressed a somewhat similar view, when he wrote:

"Sleep is a death, whereby we live a middle moderating point between life and death, and so like death, I dare not trust it without my prayers and a half adieu unto the world, and take my farewell in a colloquy with God, after which I close my eyes in security, content to take my leave of him and sleep unto the resurrection."

> "As a goldsmith, taking a piece of gold, turns it into another, newer and more beautiful shape, even so does the self, after having thrown away this body and dispelled its ignorance, make unto himself another . . ."
>
> —*Brihad-aranyaka Upanishad*

14. *The law of return*

The doctrine of rebirth, commonly called reincarnation, is no longer the prodigy it once was in the West.

In recent years the subject has been popularized by lecturers, religious teachers, and a great number of books that have appeared.

Also, in the wake of the controversial Bridey Murphy story, hypnotists—drawing room and professional—have probed the mysteries of regression, often with contradictory results.

Under the pressure of questioning by their lay members, clergymen of various faiths have had to re-examine their respective theologies to see what, if anything, they have to say about the idea of pre-existence.

Doctrine of rebirth

Roman Catholics, as well as the more orthodox and conservative Christian bodies, reject the idea of a soul's returning to earth in a succession of lives, probably because such a concept conflicts with the doctrine of redemption and bodily resurrection.

A number of liberal Protestant thinkers, on the other hand, have found the case for reincarnation a compelling one, not unsupported by their own scripture.

They point to passages in both the Old and New Testaments which seem to imply a belief in palingenesis.

For example, in the book of Malachi, the prophet declares:

"Behold, I will send you Elijah the prophet before the coming of the great and terrible day of the Lord."

At the time Malachi wrote his prophecy, Elijah had been dead many years. Therefore, it could be assumed that he might reincarnate again.

Later, in the New Testament (Matthew XVI:13), the disciples tell Jesus that some of the people think he is Elijah; others that he is John the Baptist come back; still others, that he is Jeremiah or one of the other prophets returned in another body.

Again, in St. John's Gospel (IX:34), the disciples ask Jesus concerning a certain blind man, whether his affliction was the result of some sin he had committed in a former life.

Even Catholic churchmen have not been unanimous in repudiating belief in all forms of rebirth. Belgian Cardinal Mercier, for one, declared that with respect to the assumption that the soul returns to earth many times and maintains consciousness of its personality, "We do not see that reason, if left to itself, would declare this to be impossible or certainly false."

Another Catholic prelate who reportedly accepted the doctrine of reincarnation and asserted that such a belief did not conflict with the dogma of the Church, was Archbishop Passavalli of Italy (d. 1897).

Some of the Church Fathers of the first centuries of the Christian era believed in pre-existence of the Soul, and several (like Justin Martyr and Annobius) apparently believed in a theory of palingenesis similar to that held by the Hindus.

A small number of these early Christian mystics reconciled the seeming paradox of many lives and a single resurrection of the body by declaring that the resurrected body of the "last days" would be a composite of those lived before.

Despite the Church's official opposition to the belief in reincarnation, the doctrine continued to flourish among secret and heretical Christian sects.

In this class must certainly be included such groups as the Manicheans, the Priscillians in Spain; the Cathars who numbered among their members the ill-fated Waldensians of France; the Paulicians of Armenia; and the Transcendentalists of Germany.

To trace the history of the doctrine of rebirth back to its original source is almost impossible. If vanished continents such as Atlantis and Lemuria did exist, it probably was first taught there. It is said that death as we know it was unknown until man fell from his high estate.

Be that as it may, the belief in reincarnation and karma appeared in India at an early date. It is referred to in the Atharva Veda, the Laws of Manu, the Bhagavat Purana, and in the various Upanishads.

In the sixth century B.C., it became a fundamental tenet of Buddhism. And with that faith it spread to China, Tibet, Ceylon, Burma, Indo-China, Korea and Japan.

Among the ancient Greeks, belief in reincarnation made its appearance first among the mystery schools, such as that of Orpheus, which no doubt had received it from Indian sources.

It passed quickly from religious doctrine into the area of philosophy, where it was taught by such eminent thinkers as Pythagoras, Socrates, Plato, Empedocles, and Heraclitus.

The Romans, to whom so much of the Greek philosophical heritage commended itself, gave serious thought to the concept of multiple earthly lives. Among those supporting it were Cicero, Seneca, Ovid, Virgil and Sallust. The Emperor Julian believed himself to be a reincarnation of Alexander the Great. And the poet Ennius said it had been revealed to him that he had lived before as Homer, the immortal bard of Greece.

There is, in fact, a long and impressive roster of prominent thinkers and literati who have embraced the concept in modern times. They include philosophers Giordano Bruno, Leibnitz, Hume, Lessing, Schlegel, Fichte, Herder, Schopenhauer and Emerson.

Among artists, to mention but a few, there are such diverse figures as Shelley, Wordsworth, Tennyson, Browning, Whitman, Longfellow; Wagner, Mahler; Salvador Dali, Henry Ford, Benjamin Franklin, and others.

Despite its long and honorable history, however, the deeper implications and meaning of rebirth are only vaguely understood by people in the West today.

The questions that most commonly arise are: If I have lived before, why do I not remember anything of my past lives? Why does the soul re-enter another physical body when it is often so glad to be free of the whole miserable mess on earth?

For an adequate answer to these queries, it is necessary first to direct one's attention to the nature and history of the permanent entity that is believed to reincarnate—the soul.

Westerners, when they think of the soul at all, loosely imagine some immaterial, formless luminosity; or a kind of etheric, spiritualized double of individualized man. Asked to define soul, persons of any given group—even of the same religious denomination—would present a surprising variety of descriptions.

This is quite to be expected in view of the fact that theologians themselves have provided confused and often contradictory opinions concerning the matter.

From earliest times, Christian exegetes have discussed the soul at great length without actually defining it in an easy-to-grasp, concrete way. Instead, they have referred to it in such abstract terms as incorporeal, mutable, imperishable, volitional, cognitive, and so on.

"If you wish a definition of what the soul is," wrote St. Augustine, "I have a ready answer. It seems to me to be a certain kind of substance, sharing in reason, fitted to rule the body."

But one cannot help wondering what *kind* of substance—a wraithlike vapor, a gob of ectoplasm, a ray of light, a sub-atomic particle? The theologians do not venture to say.

The ancient Hindu sages, on the other hand, were never afraid to come to grips with such mystical problems. They gave the soul size and appearance—something you could envision within the framework of human apperception.

The soul, declares the Katha Upanishad (II.13), is a *person,* compressed in form to the size of one's thumb, who dwells in the middle of the body (the heart) "like a smokeless flame. He is the lord of the past and the future. He is the same today and the same tomorrow."

Moreover, the sacred text informs us, this individual self, "that person who is awake in those that sleep," is wholly separate from physical man. If man loses his soul, he disintegrates, ceases to exist. But the soul can exist without man.

What then, is the purpose of incarnation? Why does the soul, being of its own nature free, deathless and transcendent, imprison itself within human flesh, which is conditioned; and which suffers and dies?

Tantrik method of knowing past lives

The Tantrik answer to this question is that souls enter earthly embodiment and undertake physical experience in order to achieve a divine purpose. The immediate and motivating cause of return to earth is desire, born of the past life.

But the soul's fleshly counterpart is primarily an instrument of service to a higher being. Only by becoming one with this Golden Person in the heart can the individualized self come to know all that the soul's memory holds from the past.

According to the Indian view, in each incarnation the soul assumes a different physical consciousness, a different mind and body.

The reason for this succession of mortal identities is that various types of personality and form are necessary for the soul to accomplish its mission, which is to extend God's plan of creative development to its ultimate fulfillment.

At the same time, none of these individual entities is permanently lost. For each has its archetype in the akashic records, which are eternal.

Also, firmly rooted in the heart of each of us is the memory of the loves, griefs, friendships and enmities of our former lives. It is for this reason that the haunting fragment of a song, a certain facade or doorway in the evening light, the face of a stranger upon first meeting sometimes unaccountably stir within us joyous or uneasy feelings.

Yet, is nothing more than these uncertain intimations of our long past available to us? Must we satisfy ourselves with merely fleeting, poignant impressions of those former beings for whose actions in some lost and forgotten day and place we must today suffer or exalt?

The Tantrik answer is yes and no.

Yogis who have achieved that high state of consciousness known as enlightenment have said they could, at will, recall in totality all the incarnations that had gone before.

Gautama Buddha told his disciples in detail of five hundred and fifty former lives.

And in the celebrated Hindu scripture, the Bhagavad Gita, Lord Krishna tells Arjuna:

"Both you and I have passed through many births. You know them not; I know them all."

Thus, to those great sages who have attained final union with their souls, that immortal being's storehouse of memory is thrown open to them.

But for most of us, aside from rare cases which must be regarded as abnormal, previous existences are like lost dreams. At best we can only hope to recover brief scenes or fragmentary idyls that often haunt us like a spirit.

Those who have mastered the secrets of deepest Tantrik sadhana assure us that such waking amnesia is a blessing in disguise. Only because we are free of those places, people and things of the past, which held us in bondage, can we create anew our countless individual worlds that hang like two billion dew drops in the Web of Brahma.

Of course, the residue of experience incurred in past lives remains. Unconsciously we draw upon it in myriad ways. It manifests itself as talent or innate abilities; it secretly determines many of our tastes and traits of character, erroneouly attributed to heredity or environment.

Knowing, therefore, that the sadhaka will surely in this life eat of the fruit—good and bad—of past existences, Tantrik gurus do not ordinarily teach him to resurrect, so to speak, the long succession of individual entities which, in sum, make him what he is today.

"The soul is nourished by its entire history," said Pundit Chatterjee. But we need examine particular details only when a problem has persisted from life to life.

"You should not dip into your past as into the grave. There you will find only bones and a shroud.

"Instead, let the sadhaka try to recover only those personalities and events which registered most strongly in the soul's memory because they translated the will of God into thought and deed. They are preserved in the *anahata* center, in the depth of the human heart.

"By depersonalizing his present body through a process of mantra and meditation, the yogi will surely see past embodiments emerge from the mirror-sphere of existence."

SEVENTH DISCIPLINE

Sit erect upon a chair in front of a mirror large enough to reflect your head and shoulders. A lighted candle should be placed beside the mirror in such a way that it illuminates the glass, but is not reflected in it. There should be no other light in the room.

After a moment of complete relaxation, in which you try to withdraw consciousness into your self, begin to breathe gently and rhythmically to the 7:1:7:1 count employed in previous disciplines.

Perform twelve complete cycles of this pranayama. Then remain a moment or two in *nishta*—that is, breathing very softly through both nostrils, never filling the lungs more than one eighth full.

Now form the "mudra of integration" with the right

hand, by closing the last two fingers and folding the thumb down across them, leaving the middle and index fingers outstretched.

Place the hand, held in this mudra, palm-down over the heart, the two outstretched fingers pointing toward the left side of the body.

As the heart-beat is felt beneath this hand, mentally repeat the seed syllables OM and HUM with each throb. That is to say, OM would be joined to the systolic pulsation, and HUM to the diastolic. However, it is not necessary to be too exacting. Simply join OM to one beat and HUM to the next.

These syllables are said to open the heart, permitting the sadhaka to enter it. Repeat them twenty-one times. Then close your eyes.

Form the left hand into the same mudra as that of the right. With it, cover the right hand. Then slowly withdraw the right hand, leaving the left in its place over the heart. The extended two fingers of the left hand will, of course, be pointing in the opposite direction, toward the right side of the body.

With eyes still closed, imagine your consciousness penetrating the interior of the heart. It is visualized as an arched cavern, filled at first with billowing clouds of red mist. Gradually these part and a radiant figure appears, surrounded by an aura of golden light.

Mentally, you seek to commune with this luminous being (which is your deepest self). To it you fervently address your petition for a deeper understanding, a momentary glimpse into the timeless mystery of being and becoming.

As you thus meditate in profound silence and rapture, the Golden Person dissolves once more into the red mist. But now the cavern vibrates to a chiming note of pure mantric sound, which gradually merges into silence.

The left-hand mudra is now replaced with the right one once more, reversing the procedure previously followed.

This done, open your eyes. Gaze earnestly, but with detachment, at your reflection in the mirror. This should be done without blinking or moving the eyes.

Presently, as you stare steadily into the mirror, you will see your image dissolve or disappear suddenly. You will be looking at an empty glass.

Do not start to reason about this, nor allow your gaze to waver. If you persevere, another face (sometimes a succession of faces) will supersede the familiar visage you are accustomed to seeing when you look into a mirror.

The new face will be the likeness of one of your past lives upon earth. Study it carefully. Leave your mind open to the intuitive awareness of its message and connection with your present embodiment.

When the eyes begin to fill with tears, terminate the discipline by simply intoning the syllable OM, drawing it out until the final vibration is inaudible.

In practicing this discipline, the sadhaka is urged to bear in mind that its purpose is not to satisfy idle curiosity. Rather, it is used for healing of the mind and body by a moment's revelation, which overcomes temporality and lays bare to him the eternal present.

That moment vanishes, but its all-illuminating power endures.

> "Artabhaga, my dear, take my hand. We two alone shall know of this; this is not for us two to discuss in public."
>
> —*Brihad-aranyaka Upanishad*

15. *Epilogue*

In the preceding chapters, we have taken the reader as far along the secret trail of Tantrism as he dare go without the personal supervision of a guru.

There may even be those who will argue that we have already gone too far.

We would answer these critics by recalling once again the Tantrik view that in the final analysis there is but one guru for all men, and that is God Himself. When the human guru initiates the disciple, he is only an instrument of the Supreme Guide.

"He it is who dwells within and speaks with the voice of the earthly guru." [1]

If the Mahakala is, indeed, the initiator and spiritual teacher of all mankind, then it was surely He who determined how much of the Tantrik doctrine and techniques should be revealed in the present work.

In conclusion, it might be well to look back briefly over the territory covered, thereby viewing Tantrism as a whole in a clearer perspective.

From the outset, it must be clear that the secret force used in Tantrik sadhana is essentially the universal power inherent in the union of opposite, but complementary, poles.

These opposites are two aspects of the same, single reality. The male aspect, called *purusha,* is pure, unmanifested consciousness. The female aspect, known as *prakriti,* and incarnated in Shakti (which is to say, in every woman), is the supreme, primal energy, the power of becoming.

Neither of the two can exist without the other. Without his Shakti or consort, Shiva (the Supreme Self) would be Shava—a corpse. And Shakti, apart from the cosmic consciousness, the static pole (Mt. Meru) of Shiva, would be uncontrolled, blind force.

From their union, "the play of Kali upon the bosom of Shiva," is born everything in the universe.

Such is the profound meaning of those Tantrik images encountered in Tibet, showing Shiva locked in an erotic embrace with his consort, Tara. The latter, oblivious of all else, gazes eternally into his eyes, as they

1 Yogini Tantra.

enact the divine drama of the world, a play that has no beginning and no end.

On the human level, the ecstasy experienced by the sadhaka in union with his shakti recapitulates in less degree that cosmic bliss.

Through the intensity of embrace, the yogi transcends the human state. The *maithuna* couple become as a single principle of being. They return to the latent condition of Brahman, wherein there is Atmarama or play of the self with the self.

But to achieve this supreme experience, a long and patient apprenticeship is necessary. It is a novitiate that calls for a gradual intensifying of the senses, rather than a diminution of them.

To that end, Tantrik disciplines seek not only to awaken the subtle centers, but to purify and to open the psychic channels, allowing a free influx of energy from the higher planes.

Thus, the meaning of sadhana or yogic practice is twofold. It consists of awakening and unfolding forces that lie dormant within the body; and of obtaining power from the Supreme Shakti, who is manifesting through all action in the universe.

This epiphany is expressed as sound, color, scent and form, together with the interplay of forces between them. For the Tantrik, birth and death are not two separated and distant points in time, but a continuous, eternal process.

We are constantly changing, dying, and being reborn every minute. To experience the ultimate reality behind this molecular "dance of Shakti" the aspirant must find the means of transcending it, of identifying himself with the formless bliss out of which it issues.

But since the human consciousness, manifesting as mind, can not join itself to that which is formless, a *murti* or form is necessary. That *murti* is Shakti Herself.

It is for this reason that Tantriks proclaim the divinity in woman. She embodies, in microcosm, all that the Mother Power comprehends—the three qualities of created nature (gunas), which make all action possible. She becomes an instrument for realization of the spirit.

Hence, all intercourse with her, even as the most casual relationship between man and wife, lover and mistress, should be regarded as sacramental in nature.

Such an idea will seem far-fetched, indeed, to the Western mind. And the materialist will reject it, because he perceives only *sthula* or gross form, and only spirit can know spirit. He will accuse the Tantrik, as Henry Miller accused D. H. Lawrence, of trying "to build a Taj Mahal around something as simple as a good f———."

For, despite its obsession with the subject, occidental society has learned very little of the power and inner meaning of the man-woman relationship.

Even on the "safe" ground of biological sciences, some aspects of the function and effects of coition are not fully understood.

There is, for example, the curious phenomenon called telegony—the adaptation of the female organism to that of the male.

Some years ago, Dr. Jules Goldschmidt of France put forward the theory that male generative cells not only fertilize the ovum of the female, but modify her blood chemistry.

He said the millions of spermatazoa not needed for fecundation are not lost in dissolution. Instead, activated as they are by flagella, they easily penetrate the mucous membrane of the uterus and, passing through the lymphatic and blood capillaries, enter the blood stream.

"A peculiar example of telegony," he wrote, "presents itself when a white woman, who has at first lived with a Negro and afterwards with a man of her own race, presents her second husband or lover with a more or less intensely colored child. Such cases have given rise to dramatic and even tragic scenes, when the innocent woman was simply modified (telegonized) by her first cohabitant."

Dr. Goldschmidt's premise clearly suggests that, even on the physical plane, there are profound truths remaining to be discovered in the realm of sex. Evidently the Biblical assertion that the twain shall become one flesh has, like most scriptural statements, deeper meaning than has been realized.

The Tantrik is not to be denigrated, therefore, if he finds in woman and her mysteries, the means of liberation from the fetters of worldly bondage. For his is not the path of renunciation. He seeks, rather, deliverance through love and through actual experience.

"Love," declares an unpublished treatise, "can only be found by giving it; and understanding only by living it."

Rituals may differ between school and school, between East and West, but the common ground and basic constant for all must be reintegration of the two poles of being. In our darkening age of Kali, there is no other way.

"Between the poles of the conscious and the unconscious," sang Kabir, "there has the mind made a swing.

Thereon hang all beings and all worlds, and that swing never ceases its sway."

The swing is experience, the release of life force through the creative functions of living. Confusions that veil the physical mind can be pierced only by living truth, not by reasoning about it.

Only from experience can come the realization that, in reality, nothing in this world of *samsara* (created form) is what it seems to be. Finding the source of his fears to be a delusion of worldly life, one transcends them. He can then laugh at having been frightened by "a tiger in a dream."

For every man, whether he wills it so or not, life itself is a sadhana. Until he fulfills the mission that brought him into the world, he will not be free of it and he will return to it.

The drama of the world is enacted with the rhythm and the cadence of a song. Some sing it well. Others never learn its meaning and therefore never find its melody.

Appendix
Doctrine of the vital airs

The safe and successful practice of Tantrism requires a carefully laid yogic foundation. Without such preparation, gurus warn that certain dangers may lurk along the way for the unwary. At best, they say, the sadhana will not bear fruit.

This is especially true as regards the central discipline of Shaktism, the Panchatattva or Secret Ritual. It is, indeed, for this reason that there are constant reminders in the sacred texts of the importance of that prime requirement known as *adhikara*—the aspirant's spiritual capacity or competence to practice.

As explained in earlier chapters of the present work, the practice of Tantra Yoga begins with a cleansing of the *nadis* or mystic ducts through which must flow vital currents from the subtle body or so-called "etheric double," into the gross physical organism.

Purification of these psychic channels, and stimulation of the centers of radiation (chakras) from which they emanate, is accomplished by means of breathing exercises.

Yogic breath control, of course, is not aimed solely at increasing the oxygen content of the blood, as in the case of deep-breathing exercises performed in Western gymnasiums.

Its objective is, rather, the absorption and distribution throughout the system, of that cosmic life force known as prana. It is for this reason that breath regulation techniques are called pranayama, meaning control of prana, not of breath per se.

Whatever other differences exist among the methods of the various Tantrik schools, all of them agree as to the importance of pranayama as a necessary means of purification required for *diksha* or initiation. The Gautamiya Tantra, for example, declares:

"O man of good life! there is no principle, no austerity, knowledge, state, yoga, treasure or other thing superior to pranayama . . . There is no path to liberation without pranayama, so that whatever sadhana is performed without pranayama becomes fruitless.

Prana, the universal *elan vital,* enters the human entity through the psychic centers. Thereafter it is modified according to function and location within the body.

Five of these modifications or modalities, known as *vayus* or "vital airs," are important to the Tantrik practitioner. The first and principal "air" is known by the same designation as the solar breath itself—that is, as prana. It manifests itself on the physical level as hangsah or the continuing act of respiration within the animal body.

According to some texts, its activity is centered in the region of the anahat chakra or cardiac plexus. Clairvoyants perceive it as a golden radiance, like diffused sunlight.

The remaining four airs and their functions are:

Apana, called the "downward breath," is the vital air which circulates through the muladhara or root chakra, situated between the anus and the genitals. It controls nutrition and excretion in the gross body. Some authorities say that the *apana* air is expelled *from* the body just as prana is drawn into it from a circumambient supply. It has, therefore the nature of a waste product, like carbon dioxide, expelled from the lungs. To psychic sight, it appears to be various shades of red, depending upon the individual and other circumstances.

Samana, working through the manipura or navel center, stokes the body's fires, as it were, and governs the process of digestion. It has been described by those having psychic vision as being sometimes cloudy white, sometimes of a greenish hue.

Udana, whose point of focus is the vishuddha or throat chakra, regulates the functioning of the diaphragm, thereby influencing the rhythm and depth of respiration. At the time of death, it also acts to release the subtle body from the hold of the gross one. A familiar manifestation of this separation of the physical from the non-physical is the peculiar sound in the throat sometimes referred to as "the death rattle." To esoteric perception, the *udana* current is pale blue.

Vayana is a dynamic, operative current, which pervades the entire body, vitalizing tissues and controlling circulation of blood. It is said to have as its point of emanation the swadisthana chakra at the root of the genitals. Its color varies from lucent rose in a person who enjoys good health, to a pale pink in an enfeebled or diseased organism.

Defining the function of the vital airs in a somewhat broader sense, one Tantrik work says that prana is the power of appropriation; *apana* that of rejection; *samana*, of assimilation; *udana* of articulation; and *vayana* of distribution.

This specialized activity of the vital airs is, of course, involuntary so far as the animal organism is concerned, but its strength and scope can be intensified and expanded by voluntary effort.

Each cycle of respiration in every individual reacts dynamically upon the static coiled power at the base of the cerebro-spinal axis—the kundalini. It is a reaction that occurs an average of 21,600 times a day, for that is the number of breaths taken by the ordinary man.

However, these breaths are shallow and fairly rapid in the case of the majority of men. They fill the lungs to only one sixth their capacity. The result is that the current of energy sent downward to strike at the coiled kundalini asleep at the root chakra does not awaken it.

Yogic breathing exercises, on the other hand, send a potent charge of prana coursing toward the kundalini. When this charge enters the area controlled by the navel center, it begins to glow like a fire fanned by a bellows.

The resulting *tumo* heat, according to the Yoga-Kundali Upanishad, arouses the dormant kundalini, which "awakens from her sleep as a serpent, struck by a stick, hisses and straightens itself." It thereupon enters the central channel of the spine (the sushumna) and starts its ascent toward the crown of the head.

Some authorities say that the serpent power thus released is an emanation rather than the mother kundalini herself. The latter, they maintain, remains coiled in the cavity near the base of the spine, merely sending forth an etheric counterpart.

As the kundalini energy proceeds up the central channel, it vitalizes each chakra and purifies the nadis related to it. When it reaches the highest center of the subtle body (the sahasrara), it unites with the maha-kundali of Shiva residing there, and polarizes every cell of the body.

The primary aim of breathing techniques is thus, obviously, to force prana—the upward breath—to flow downward and to strike the latent kundalini; and to cause the *apana* or downward breath, to rise. By reversing their usual direction and by bringing them together at the navel chakra, great psychic heat is generated.

One of the first indications (aside from heat) that the kundalini has entered the median duct and begun its ascent is that prana ceases to move in the *ida* and *pingala* nadis (left and right nostrils). Breathing appears to be suspended altogether.

The technique is not an easy one, and must be mastered gradually. It is only after considerable practice that the serpent fire will enter the sushumna passage.

Moreover, the procedure is not without its dangers. The sadhaka is especially cautioned that if pain occurs in the abdominal region, the practice should be discontinued. When such discomfort occurs, it is because the kundalini current has met with resistance at one of the three points in its upward ascent, known as *"granthis"* or "knots." They mark the juncture of the nadis with the root, cardiac and brow chakras, respectively.

The first knot is often referred to as the Knot of Brahma; the second the Knot of Vishnu; and the third, the Knot of Shiva.

The symbolism recalls a quatrain from the Rubaiyat of Omar Khayyam, one of almost certain Tantrik import:

"Up from Earth's Center through the Seventh Gate
I rose, and on the throne of Saturn sate,
*   And many a knot unravel'd by the Road*
But not the Master-Knot of Human Fate."

It will be recalled that the muladhara or root chakra is commonly called the Earth Center chakra.

Tantrik gurus warn that in the case of persons who are at certain stages of spiritual evolution, a cosmic counter force called Maya-Shakti is especially strong at the three centers mentioned. If the *sadhaka* persists in trying to force the psychic current through the "knots," physical disorders will result. It is also possible to do permanent injury to the central nervous system.

If signs of physical distress appear during practice, therefore, the disciple is strongly urged to forego further practice until such a time as he may place himself under the supervision of a competent guru.

As regards the best times of day to practice pranayama, most texts state that, unless otherwise indicated, the best hours are sunrise, noon, sunset and midnight.

Prana, like a cosmic tide, ebbs and flows in the human

body. At sunrise, it enters the sushumna canal. At noon it is equalized in the nadis and in the blood stream. At sunset, it courses through the arteries of the physical body in flood tide. At midnight it rests in the hollow of the heart and in the blood vessels, like motionless slack-water between the ocean tides.

Thus, from noon to midnight, while prana circulates with the blood, physical stamina is naturally at its peak. From midnight until noon, prana is polarized in the nerves. Consequently, during that interval, nervous energy necessary for intellectual tasks is more abundant. This may, to some extent, account for the fact that many writers and creative artists in all ages have been "night-owls," finding the post-midnight and early morning hours the best for their work.

At whatever hour circumstances may force the sa-dhaka to practice, regularity is essential. Once the disciplines are made a part of everyday routine, like bathing and taking meals, they will be easier to perform and will show quicker results.

The neophyte often asks, when is the best time to embark upon a course of exercises?

Some Tantrik authorities advise starting in the Spring or Autumn; during the moon's first quarter; and when the breath flow is through the ida or left nostril.

Additional general rules governing the practice of pranayama usually include these:

The sadhaka ought to seat himself upon a red woolen pad during practice. An ordinary blanket is satisfactory for the purpose. Many Hindu teachers hold the view that use of an uncovered wooden seat brings ill health and material loss.

Mental attitude is also important. Practice should be

initiated with the positive thought that it will produce the desired results. It helps tremendously to "get into the mood," as it does in the case of most undertakings which require concentration and skill. Reading of yogic texts is one way of inducing such a state of mind. The role of will power (called yoga-bala) is emphasized by almost all Tantrik schools. Many of them employ images and mystic diagrams to help create the proper frame of mind.

Breathing exercises should never be undertaken on a full stomach; when the sadhaka is tired or ill; nor immediately following violent physical exertion.

A little butter dissolved in the mouth just prior to starting pranayama will lubricate the throat for passage of air during measured respiration.

When practice is indoors, the room must be well-ventilated, cheerful, dry, and free of dust and noise.

With the foregoing rationale and rules of practice clearly in mind, the student is ready to proceed with the graded series of exercises which follow in the proper sequence.

First discipline: eight weeks

FIRST WEEK

Time: Morning.
Place: Well-ventilated room.
Duration: Twelve times.
Technique: Assume the posture you have found

most suitable for practice, spine straight, chin in a straight line with the chest.

For a moment, try to relax completely, emptying the mind of all cares and trivial thoughts. Expel all air from the lungs by sharply drawing in the abdomen as you exhale.

Slowly refill the lungs to the count of seven. Pause for one count, then exhale to the count of seven again. This cycle should be repeated twelve times to establish smooth, rhythmic, deep respiration.

Now exhale through both nostrils to fill the lungs as full as possible without discomfort. Hold the breath in the mouth, forcing it against the cheeks until they bulge. Retain the breath this way as long as it is comfortable to do so. Then expel it quickly and explosively through the mouth, once more using the abdominal muscles to force out all the air.

Repeat the procedure, mentally reciting the mantram OM as you inhale. In your imagination, picture a pulsating current of life force flowing into your lungs with the breath. Then envision this vital stream flowing like divine ichor through the spreading web of nadis or psychic channels of the subtle body and thence into the physical organism, energizing every cell.

The foregoing cycle should be repeated twelve times at each sitting.

SECOND WEEK

Time: Sunrise or at sunset.
Place: Open country, park, seashore, mountain trail, desert or woods.

Duration: Twelve times, twice daily.

Technique: If possible, go for a walk before breakfast and again before dinner in the evening, preferably in the country or through a park.

Your pace should be leisurely and your mind free of insistent cares that ordinarily make you tense or apprehensive of the future. As you stroll along, slowly inhale through both nostrils to the count of seven. Retain the breath for two counts. Then exhale through the mouth to the count of seven. Hold the breath outside for two counts. Repeat the cycle twelve times.

After practicing three days, increase the ratio from 7:2:7:2 to 10:5:10:5.

If you do not find it convenient to practice morning and evening, you may perform the sadhana at any time during the day or night. A solitary walk is, however, necessary.

THIRD WEEK

Time: Morning and evening.

Place: Well-ventilated room or secluded place outdoors.

Duration: Twenty-four times, twice daily.

Technique: Seated in the comfortable posture customarily assumed for sadhana, purse the lips as when pronouncing the syllable "oo." Inhale through the mouth with the lips in this position, seven small draughts. Then swallow. Exhale through both nostrils, again to the count of seven. Repeat the cycle twenty-four times morning and evening.

Time: Optional; but practice should be at the same hour every day.

Place: Well-ventilated room or secluded place outdoors.

Duration: Twelve times.

Technique: Seated in the meditative posture, facing the direction of the sun, equalize the respiratory rhythm by breathing slowly in and out to the measure 7:1:7:1, as described in previous disciplines.

After a few moments, when deep, rhythmic breathing has been established, inhale through both nostrils to the count of four or until the lungs are about half filled. Then, holding the breath, curl the tongue backward as far as possible against the roof of the mouth. Holding it thus, emit a loud growl: "Grrrr!" as you exhale.

FIFTH WEEK

Time: Morning and noon.

Place: Outdoors or near an open window.

Duration: Six times.

Technique: Standing with the feet apart to form a V, softly whistle a few bars of some familiar song. Keeping the lips puckered, inhale slowly through the mouth to the count of seven. Pause for a single count. Then exhale through both nostrils to the count of seven. Repeat this cycle six times in the morning and six times at noon.

Time: Morning, noon and evening.

Place: Well-ventilated room or secluded place out-doors.

Duration: Five times.

Technique: Standing with the feet apart, as in the preceding exercise; or seated in the customary posture for sadhana, face the sun. After equalizing the breath by breathing slowly in and out to the 7:1:7:1 rhythm, place the tongue between the lips and protrude it slightly. Draw air into the lungs through the mouth with a hissing sound. When the lungs are filled, retain the breath as long as possible without discomfort. Then exhale gently through both nostrils. Repeat the cycle five times. Practice it morning, noon, and evening for two weeks.

Students who are being treated for an overactive thyroid should omit this exercise altogether. Conversely, those suffering from hypothyroidism should perform it twice the prescribed number of times.

EIGHTH WEEK

Time: Sunrise

Place: Near an open window or in a secluded place out of doors.

Duration: Five to twelve times.

Technique: Seated in the customary posture of sadhana, force all the air from the lungs by vigorously exhaling while drawing in the abdominal wall.

Now close the right nostril with the right thumb, and slowly exhale through the left nostril to the count of four. Close both nostrils and retain the breath for a count of sixteen. Then, keeping the left nostril closed, exhale through the right to the count of eight. Still keeping the left nostril closed, inhale through the right for four counts; again retain sixteen; and, closing the right nostril, exhale through the left for eight counts.

For the first three days of practice, repeat the cycle five times. On the succeeding four days, increase the number of cycles to twelve.

Second discipline: ninth week

Time: Between 9:30 a.m. and noon.
Place: Before an open window, in full sunlight.
Duration: Three times for each color.
Technique: Assume the posture for sadhana, facing East. Close the eyes, and for a brief time visualize the radiant energy of the sun entering your subtle and gross bodies to permeate and vitalize every cell.

Sit upright and empty the lungs, forcing out residual air in the manner previously described. Then slowly inhale to the count of seven. Retain the breath for seven counts, meanwhile strongly visualizing the color red. Direct the consciousness to the lower portion of the stomach and genitals, and imagine a flood of red light covering that area of your body.

Exhale to the count of seven. Pause one count, then repeat the red cycle. Perform it three times.

Follow the same procedure and measurement of time intervals for yellow. Mentally picture a deluge of effulgent yellow light bathing the region of the upper chest and forehead.

Repeat the exercise with blue. Visualize that color spreading over the throat area, solar plexus, and crown of the head in a cool, healing, spiritual radiance.

After three cycles of this color, pause one second. Then perform the same pranayama, suffusing the feet, legs, arms and face with awareness of pure white light.

During the last four days that this discipline is practiced, perform the sadhana at midnight, as well as in the hours before noon.

Third discipline: tenth week

Time: Hours between midnight and dawn.
Place: A secluded place where there is a minimum of sound and where you will not be interrupted.
Duration: Fifteen minutes daily.
Technique: Seated in sadhana posture, face either East or North. Perform *japa mantra* by breathing in and out rhythmically, joining to the respiration the mental repetition of the mystic syllable OM. Inhalation is to the count of seven; one count between breaths; and exhalation to the count of seven. If you find it difficult to count and to repeat the syllable at the same time, repetition of the syllable is more important.

The syllable is repeated one hundred and eight times with the incoming and outgoing breaths. To keep count of the breath cycles, a rosary of one hundred and eight beads should be used. The rosary should be of pearls, crystals, gold, silver, coral, or of *rudraksha* seeds.

After recitation of the syllable OM, sit quietly, gazing steadily and without blinking, at some fixed point (e.g., a candle flame) on level with the eyes and at a distance of about five feet. While focusing the attention on this point, listen intently with the right ear for the inner sound. It may be perceived in one of a variety of ways—as tiny silver chains, humming bees, bells, a flute, ocean roar, etc., as enumerated in Chapter 6.

If the sound is not heard by the third day of practice, perform the folowing exercise:

Seated in sadhana posture, facing East, rest the elbows on a pillow placed in front of you upon a desk or table. Place the thumbs lightly upon the small flaps of the ears and press them to close the ears to outside sounds. Close the eyes and place the index fingers on the lids; the middle fingers and ring fingers should press the lids between them.

Breathe rhythmically but slowly in and out through both nostrils. Meanwhile, direct the consciousness to the closed ears, listening in an attentive but detached way, for the sounds to be heard within.

Fourth discipline: eleventh week

Time: Preferably between 7 p.m. and midnight.
Place: Clean, well-ventilated room, affording complete privacy and freedom from interruption.

Duration: Pranayama—twelve times; *maithuna*—a minimum of thirty-two minutes.

Technique: Following a bath, enter the practice room and light the ritual candles. Assume the posture of sadhana. Empty the lungs of residual air, as in preceding disciplines. Equalize the breath by breathing rhythmically in and out to the 7:1:7:1 ratio. Complete twelve cycles of this rhythm. Then, upon drawing in the thirteenth breath, retain it for a count of seven before exhaling—again, to seven counts. During the retention (*kumbhak*) concentrate intently upon the root chakra, situated between the anus and genitals.

Mentally picture a current of prana flowing to the center. Stimulate it physically by contracting the sphincter muscles of the anus. As this is being done, envision a psychic current rising upward through the central channel of the spine to the crown of the head. The retention cycle is also repeated twelve times.

Thereafter the sadhaka proceeds with the secret ritual, as described in Chapter 9.

Fifth discipline: twelfth week

Time: Optional.

Place: Secluded, but well-ventilated room.

Duration: Preparatory phase—twelve cycles. Second phase—two minutes. Final phase—three to seven times.

Technique: Seated upon a woolen pad in sadhana

posture, face the East. Equalize the breath by breathing slowly and deeply in and out to the 7:1:7:1 count used in previous disciplines. Repeat the cycle twelve times. Then relax, allowing the breath to flow on of its own accord.

After a moment or two of complete tranquility, grasp the left wrist and upper portion of the left hand (back side) with the right hand. With hands thus joined, place them palms downward over the transformation center at the solar plexus.

Close the eyes and mentally picture within this center a small, brilliant tongue of flame, hair-thin and twisted at the top like a corkscrew.

Once this image has been clearly formed in the mind's eye, again equalize the breath with the 7:1:7:1 rhythm. As the breath flows in and out, imagine that it fans the glowing tongue of flame within the solar center, heating it to white-hot incandescence.

As you begin to feel a kindling warmth in the area of the solar plexus, substitute for the flame image a mental picture of the thing or condition you wish to materialize on the physical plane.

When you have clearly pictured the object or condition you desire, draw the abdominal wall back and forth spasmodically, so that the breath will come and go in staccato spurts. Continue this phase of the sadhana for two minutes, all the while visualizing your objective and strongly willing it to materialize.

Then lower the head until the chin rests firmly against the chest. Expel all air from the lungs. Hold the breath outside the lungs for a count of seven. With hands still clasped in the mudra described above, press against the solar plexus, meanwhile trying to agitate that area with a quick, vibrating motion. Again bring into sharp mental focus a visualization of the thing you desire.

Inhale once more, raising the head upward until you are gazing at the ceiling of the room. Then, locking the breath within, force the air downward until it is felt pressing against the diaphragm.

Retain the breath thus for seven counts. As you do so, picture the *tumo* fire again entering the central canal of the spine and passing upward toward the Brahma-randhra or crown of the head. Mentally affirm that as the serpent fire rises, it carries with it the substance of your desire.

Exhale, visualizing the desire as now being outside yourself—an objective, free-moving, vitalized thought form.

Sixth discipline: thirteenth week

Time: When retiring for the night.

Place: A quiet, pleasantly appointed bedroom.

Duration: The time necessary to pass from the wak-ing state (jagrat) to that of sleep (svapna).

Technique: After retiring for the night, and with the lights extinguished, lie upon your back in bed, hands clasped in the mudra of the preceding dis-cipline. Rest the hands over the solar plexus.

Lie quietly for a few moments, relaxing in mind and body. Equalize the breath with the 7:1:7:1 rhythm for twelve cycles. Then turn and lie upon the right side;

pull the legs slightly upward until the knees are bent to relieve tension in the legs. Rest the left arm outstretched along the left leg. Cup the palm of the right hand and rest the right cheek in it.

Join the syllable OM to the breath flow, strongly resolving to retain memory and awareness through the dream state.

For those phases of this discipline other than pranayama, review the procedure outlined in Chapter 13 on Yoga of the Dream State.

Seventh discipline: fourteenth week

Time: Sunset to midnight.

Place: Secluded room, affording complete privacy.

Duration: First phase—twelve cycles. Second phase —twenty-one times.

Technique: Sit erect in a straight chair, before a mirror sufficiently large to reflect your head and shoulders. Place a lighted candle to the right of the mirror in a position that illuminates the glass, without reflecting an image of the candle. Extinguish all other lights in the room.

For a few moments sit quietly, allowing the thoughts to flow as they will, without taking any of them up consciously. Then equalize the breath by means of the 7:1:7:1 rhythm. Repeat the cycle twelve times, then inhale gently through both nostrils only enough air to fill the lungs to about one-eighth their capacity.

Close the small and ring fingers of the right hand into

the palm, and fold the thumb down across them, leaving the middle and index fingers outstretched.

Place the hand palm downward over the cardiac region of the chest, the two outstretched fingers pointing toward the left side of the body.

As the heart throb is felt beneath the hand, mentally repeat the syllables OM and HUM alternately with the heartbeats. Repeat the syllables twenty-one times (forty-two counts in all), then form the left hand into a mudra similar to that just executed with the right. Cover the right hand with the left, then slowly withdraw the right, leaving the left in its place over the heart, fingers now pointing toward the right side of the body.

With eyes closed, try to penetrate the interior of the heart. Visualize an arched, dimly lighted cavern, filled with clouds of red mist. Gradually the swirling vapor clouds part and a figure clothed in bright golden light emerges.

Still breathing lightly but rhythmically, focus your deepest thought and aspirations upon this luminous figure. Mentally address to it your wordless longing for contact with your soul's lost identities. Say to it:

"Reveal, reveal thyself to me."

Wait in profound silence until the golden figure is enveloped once more by the billowing red mist, and the cavern of the heart echoes a single note of pure sound, which softly dies away into silence.

Then replace the left hand with the right one. Open your eyes and earnestly regard your reflection in the mirror. After a brief moment, it will disappear, leaving an empty mirror. Continue to stare at the glass with calm detachment.

If your sadhana is successful, another face or series of

faces will appear in the glass. Study them objectively and, if possible, without emotion, seeking to learn what they have to reveal. Avoid blinking the eyes during this phase of the discipline, if you can do so. When tears appear, conclude the sadhana by intoning the syllable OM, attenuating the sound until it merges into silence.

The exercise should not be practiced more than once in a twenty-four-hour period. However, it may and should be repeated nightly until some measure of success is achieved.

After performing the foregoing principal disciplines of purification and merging, the sadhaka may take up other practices for control of the vital breaths.

But complete mastery of Tantrik techniques should take precedence over all others.

Glossary

ADHIKARA—A disciple's competency or moral fitness to practice the secret ritual.

AGAMAS—Sacred Tantrik scripture dealing with rites, dharma, and cosmology.

AJAPA MANTRA—The involuntary prayer, "Hang-sah, Hang-sah," made by incoming and outgoing breath. It corresponds to the cosmic creative process by which the entire universe is breathed forth at intervals and then withdrawn.

AJNA—The sixth chakra or center of consciousness in the subtle body, situated between the eyebrows. It is sometimes called the Third Eye. Two wing-like "petals" or subtle channels emanate from it.

AKASHA—Ether; an invisible manifestation of primordial substance, which pervades the entire universe as its substratum.

ANAHATA—The fourth chakra or center of consciousness, situated in the cardiac region. It is sometimes called the "heart lotus." Twelve mystic ducts or "petals" emanate from it.

ASANA—Posture assumed in the practice of yoga.

BANOWA—(Tib.) The Yoga of Ascendancy, by which the yogi can influence men, animals and inanimate objects.

BARDO—(Tib.) The intermediate state of the discarnate ego, between death and rebirth.

BIJA MANTRA—A seed sound, produced from the hidden power or primordial shakti. Tantrik texts say the universe evolved out of the fifty original bija mantras, which correspond to the fifty letters of the Sanskrit alphabet.

BRAHMA-RUDHRA—The "gateway of Brahma," an aperture in the crown of the head, through which the soul may leave the body.

CHAKRAS—Six centers of consciousness and psychic energy in the subtle body. They are variously called "lotuses," "wheels," and "omphali" because of their shape. They are: the muladhara, svadhisthana, manipura, anahata, vishuddha, and ajna (q.v.).

CHITRINI—A tiny *nadi* or subtle channel for psychic current, present inside another—the *vajrini* (q.v.).

DIKSHA—Initiation by a guru.

DRAGPO—(Tib.) In Tibetan Tantrism, the wrathful or Banishing Performance by which the yogi can cause calamities, strike a person speechless, kill or destroy.

GUHYA-BHASHANAM—Intimate discussion with a person of the opposite sex.

GYAISPA—(Tib.) In Tibetan Tantrism, the power of procuring prosperity, fame, progeny, etc.

IDA—Conduit of subtle energy, coiling about the sushumna and terminating in the left nostril. Opposite in polarity from the pingala.

JITANDRIYA—Control of the senses; in Tantrism, control of the semen.

JIVATMA—The self, soul, or individual consciousness.

KANDA—In the subtle body, an egg-shaped bulb, covered with membrane; situated at a point midway between genitals and anus.

KELI—Keeping company with the opposite sex. (One of the eight subtle forms of sexual intercourse cited in Hindu texts.)

KIRTANAM—Discussing the sexual act with another; hence, one of the mental forms of coition.

KOSHA—Subtle envelope surrounding the gross body.

KRIYA-NISHPATTI—Physical sexual congress. See *maithuna*.

KUMBHAK—Retention of the breath in the practice of pranayama.

KUNDALINI—Shakti energy coiled like a sleeping serpent in a cavity near the base of the spine. When aroused by yogic discipline, or by some other means, it ascends the central channel of the spine or sushumna.

LATA-SADHANA—Tantrik discipline requiring a female consort.

LOKAS—Planes of existence inhabited by sentient beings.

MADYA—Wine, as employed in the Tantrik panchatattva or secret ritual.

MAITHUNA—Sexual union, whether symbolical or actual physical coition.

MAMSHA—Meat, one of the so-called Five M's or Five True Things used in Tantra's secret ritual.

MANIPURA—The chakra or psychic center located at the level of the solar plexus. It has ten "petals" or "spokes."

MANTRAM—Incantation. Syllables, inaudible or vocalized, used in prayer and in ritualistic formula.

MATSYA—Fish; one of the elements used in the secret ritual of Tantrism. It represents the two vital currents moving in the pingala and ida channels of the subtle body.

MOKSHA—The ultimate spiritual liberation from material bondage.

MULADHARA—The lowest of the chakras or subtle centers, situated at the base of the spine. It has four ducts emanating from it, figuratively referred to as "petals."

NADAM—Vibrational energy permeating all things, and manifesting as sound.

NADIS—Invisible conduits of psychic energy, woven throughout the subtle body "like threads in a spider web." Most authorities say there are 72,000 of them; some say 200,000 and others 350,000.

NYASA—Projection of divine entities into various parts of the body.

OJAS—Energy developed by certain yogic practices, which stimulate endocrine activity within the body.

PANCHATATTVA—Literally, the five *tattvas*. In Tantrism, it applies to the five elements or Five True Things used in the secret ritual. They are wine, fish, meat, cereal, and sexual union.

PHO-WA—(Tib.) The Yoga of Transference, known to Western occultists as astral body projection.

PINGALA—A subtle channel through which prana moves. It coils around the central sushumna canal and terminates in the right nostril. It has a positive polarity.

PRAKRITI—Manifested or materialized nature. It possesses three *gunas* or qualities, viz., *sattwa,* governing order and time; *rajas,* or activation and mental power; and *tamas,* the gross form of dense matter, characterized by stability and inertia.

PRANA—The total energy, manifest and unmanifest, of the cosmos. It is known to the earth sphere as the seven-rayed emanation from the sun. Also, the "vital air" or power behind breath.

PRANAYAMA—Yogic regulation of the breath flow for purposes of prana control.

PREKSHENAM—Flirtation.

PURAK—Inhalation process in the practice of yogic breathing.

PURUSHA—Pure, unmanifested consciousness.

RECHAK—Exhalation of air in yogic breathing exercises.

RUDRAKSHAS—Seeds of a plant used in Shiva rites, and for the 108-bead Hindu rosary.

SADHAKA—One who practices Tantrik disciplines; a yogi aspirant or disciple.

SAHASRARA—The so-called "thousand-petaled lotus," the highest subtle center of consciousness at the top of the spinal column. It is the seat of unmanifested Shiva.

SAMHITA—Mystic union, as distinct from physical coition or *maithuna* (q.v.).

SAMKALPA—A carnal desire to indulge in sexual intercourse.

SAMSARA—Created forms. Also, the world in which the law of reincarnation operates.

SANDHA-BHASA—The secret language of Tantrism.

SHABDA—Vibrational energy manifested as sound.

SHAKTI—Power; the secret force permeating all creation. Also, the divine consort of Shiva, or the ritual sexual partner of the Tantrik.

SHISHYA—Disciple or neophyte.

SHIVA—The first logos; the divine will, which manifests in creative union with Shakti.

SHIWA—(Tib.) The power to prevent misfortune befalling oneself or others.

SIDDHI—Occult or paranormal powers. They are the fruits of yogic practice, not its aim.

SMARNANAM—According to Vedic literature, one of the eight aspects of sexual intercouse, namely, allowing the thoughts to dwell upon it.

SUSHUMNA—A *nadi* or psychic channel of the subtle body, within the center of the spinal column.

SVADISTHANA—The second chakra or center of psychic radiation, situated at the root of the genitals. It has six "spokes" or "petals."

SWARA SADHANA—Practice in which the yogi causes the breath to flow through the left nostril from sunrise to sunset; and through the right nostril from sunset to sunrise.

THRONG-JUG—(Tib.) Projection of one's consciousness into, and the taking over of, another's body.

TULPA—(Tib.) Thought-form. Tibetan Tantriks are said to be able to project these mental images in the perfect likeness of men and animals and to animate them so they are mistaken for real entities.

TUMO—(Tib.) Psychic heat or mystic fire, whose seat is the Navel Chakra.

VAJRINI—A tiny duct carrying psychic energy within the subtle body, unknown to Western anatomy.

VAMACHARI—Member of a Tantrik coterie which practices certain disciplines that include the panchatattva (q.v.).

VIDYA GUPTA—Secret tradition or mystic discipline conveyed from guru to disciple only by word of mouth. It is sometimes called the "Whispered Tradition."

VISHUDDHA—The chakra or mystic center of consciousness situated at the throat level. It is also called the Great Purity center. It has sixteen "petals" of smoky purple.

YAKSHA—A female spirit or fairy; also, a guardian angel or, in Tibet, a demon.

YONI—The vulva. In Tantrik ritual it may be any symbol representing the female genitals.

YUGA—An age or vast cycle of time. The four classical yugas are: Satya yuga, Treta yuga, Dvapara yuga; and Kali Yuga, which is the present and lowest of all four.

Selected Bibliography

BAGCHI, PRABODH CHANDRA. *Studies in the Tantras.* Calcutta Sanskrit
Series, 1939.
BASU, SRI CHANDRA. *Esoteric Science and Philosophy of the Tantras.*
Allahabad: Dharma Press, 1914.
———. *Shiva Samhita,* Calcutta: 1928.
BHATTACHARYYA, BENOYTOSH. *Sadhanamala.* Gaekwar Oriental Series,
Baroda: 1928.
———. *Shanti-sangama Tantra.* Gaekwar Oriental Series, 1947.
BRAHMA, NALINTA KANTA. *The Philosophy of Hindu Sadhana.* London:
Kegan Paul, 1932.
COOMARASWAMY, ANANDA K. *Dance of Shiva,* rev. ed. New York: Noon-
day Press, 1957.
DASGUPTA, SASHI BHUSAN. *An Introduction to Tantrik Buddhism.* Cal-
cutta: University of Calcutta Press, 1950.
DAVID-NEEL, ALEXANDRA. *With Mystics and Magicians in Tibet.* New
York: University Books, 1959.

ELIADE, MIRCEA. *Yoga: Immortality and Freedom.* New York: Pantheon Books, 1958.

EVANS-WENTZ, W. Y. *The Tibetan Book of the Dead.* 3d ed. New York: Oxford University Press, 1957.

——. *Tibetan Yoga and Secret Doctrines.* 2d ed. New York: Oxford University Press, 1958.

EVOLA, GIULIO CESARE. *Lo Yoga dello Potenza.* Milan: 1949.

GOVINDA, LAMA ANAGARIKA. *Fundamentals of Tibetan Mysticism.* New York: E. P. Dutton, 1959.

JACOBS, HANS. *Western Psychotherapy and Hindu Sadhana.* International Universities Press, 1961.

PAYNE, ERNEST A. *The Shaktas.* Calcutta: 1933.

RADHAKRISHNAN, SARVEPALLI (ed.). *The Principal Upanishads.* London: Allen & Unwin, 1953.

SNELLGROVE, D. L. (ed.). *Havajra Tantra.* 2 vols. New York: Oxford University Press, 1961.

TATTVABUSHAN, HEMCHANDRA (Trans.). *Kamaratna Tantra.* Sillong: 1928.

TUCCI, GIUSEPPE. *Theory and Practice of Mandala.* New York: 1958.

——. *Indo-Tibetica.* Rome: 1932.

WOODROFFE, SIR JOHN (ARTHUR AVALON, pseud.). *The Greatness of Shiva.* Vedanta Press, 1953.

——. *The Great Liberation.* Vedanta Press, 1953.

——. *Hymns to Kali.* 2d ed. Vedanta Press, 1953.

——. *Introduction to Tantra Shastra.* 3d ed. Vedanta Press, 1956.

——. *Kamakala Vilasa.* Madras: Ganesh & Co., 1928.

——. *Kulachudamani Nigama.* 2d ed. Vedanta Press, 1956.

——. *Principles of Tantra.* Madras: Ganesh & Co., 1914.

——. *The Serpent Power.* 3d ed. Madras: Ganesh & Co., 1931.

——. *Shakti and Shakta.* Madras: Ganesh & Co., 1929.

——. *Tantraraja Tantra.* Vedanta Press, 1954.

ZIMMER, HEINRICH. *Philosophies of India.* New York: Pantheon Books, 1951.

Index